An Applicant's Guide to
Physician Assistant School and Practice

Erin L. Sherer, MPAS, PA-C, RD

An Applicant's Guide to Physician Assistant School and Practice

Printed in the United States of America.

ISBN: 1-434-82806-9

EAN-13: 978-1-4348-2806-4

Acknowledgments

This book never would have been written without the enthusiasm of my husband, who was loyal in his support and intense in his interest. His creativity, constructive criticism, and diligence in editing truly made this book possible.

I also would like to thank my colleagues in the American Association of Surgical Physician Assistants, Dan Vetrosky, MEd, PhDc, PA-C, and David DeWalch, PA-C. Both Dan and David have been incredibly supportive of this project from the beginning, and both spent a great deal of time reviewing the book and suggesting improvements.

Special thanks to my good friends, Patrick Chiu, M.D., and Kimberly Gratenstein, M.D., who also enthusiastically reviewed the project. I am grateful for all the constructive criticism and great ideas they both offered along the way.

I am also indebted to a number of current physician assistant students who helped make this book even better: Holly Morris, Danielle Belknap, Meghan Riley, Erin Lennon, Abby Bowen, and Aisha Khan. You are already accomplished professionals; by becoming physician assistants, you will make our profession even better.

And, finally, I would like to thank my parents, Jan and Chuck, and my sister, Kristin, for always supporting me in all of my personal and professional endeavors.

Table of Contents

Introduction

You might be wondering who I am, and why I am writing this book. I will begin with who I am. I have always been interested in healthcare, and my initial interests in science and health led me to the field of nutrition in college. While working as a dietitian, I then had the opportunity to watch a surgeon and physician assistant (PA) work together in the operating room. I still remember being fascinated by the interplay between the two. That fascination then formed the basis for my interest in PA school. When I considered applying, I was not sure if I would get into PA school because I knew programs were extremely competitive. So, like you, I researched the process. After carefully considering my options, and using the method I outline in this book, I applied. To my delight, I was accepted into four different physician assistant programs, including my top choice.

During my time as a PA student, I decided to take on a student leadership role within the American Association of Surgical Physician Assistants (AASPA). My experience working with AASPA inspired me to take an active role in the PA profession, and also taught me a lot about networking and leadership. As the Student Director of the AASPA, I spent nearly two years assisting PA students and pre-PA students with questions on a variety of topics, including information about the profession, obtaining PA shadowing experiences, applying for surgical residencies, obtaining PA jobs, and writing essays suitable for the Central Application Service for Physician Assistants (CASPA) submission. In addition to these duties, I also wrote articles for the student section of AASPA's journal.

As for the "why" I wrote this book, now that I have finished school and am working both as a PA and as an educator, I am still eager to help those interested in becoming a part of this profession. My previous experience assisting future PA students inspired me to share the information I learned with a broader audience. My goal with this book is simple: I want to help ambitious students gain admission into PA school programs by providing my readers with a solid background of the PA profession (how it exists today, and where it is headed tomorrow) and giving my readers skills and advice towards becoming a successful PA school applicant.

How to use this book

This book will help guide you along the process of becoming a PA. It begins by helping you, the prospective PA student, consider whether or not you really should become a physician assistant by discussing what a PA really does, and comparing the PA profession to a number of other healthcare careers. I then provide you with the necessary information to successfully apply to physician assistant educational programs. The book also provides you with information you will need to know in order to interview well, and discuss the PA profession intelligently. Finally, the book's indices provide the following: (a) further PA and prospective PA resources; (b) the minimum requirements for every PA program in the United States; and (c) current information on residencies and fellowships for PA graduates.

The chapters were written with a novice in mind, so if you read the book straight through (even if you have little or no background knowledge of the physician assistant profession), you will have no problem following the concepts. This book is organized into a series of steps which build upon one another, ultimately leading you through PA school, and on to becoming a practicing PA. While some parts of the book are quite general, others will examine specific topics related to the PA profession and the PA school application process.

This book is patterned after my own experience, and I have tried to provide concrete examples both from my own experiences working in the profession, as well as examples from other practicing clinicians. These examples will give you accurate and realistic ideas about application and practice within the profession. While some chapters may initially seem superfluous, each is important, and may help a prospective student or practicing PA when he or she least expects it. Ideally, you should read this book in its entirety before you begin applying to PA school, and use it as a reference during the PA school application process.

I hope you find this book to be both useful and enjoyable, and I wish you the best of luck as you begin your journey to successfully becoming a physician assistant.

What is a Physician Assistant?

In the PA profession, this is known as the "famous" question. What is a physician assistant, or a PA? I often find myself answering this question when it is asked in either social or clinical venues, and my response usually goes something like this:

A PA is a healthcare provider who works with a doctor. A PA can perform many of the same functions that doctors can, with or without their physical supervision. For example, we can prescribe medications, perform procedures, perform physical exams, assist in surgeries, etc…

I then try to tailor the rest of my response to the setting, giving more clinical information if I am speaking with a patient. I certainly always try to answer the question in the most "real-life" way I can, because many people working outside of healthcare have no idea what we, as PAs, do. While some PA professionals shy away from saying that our work, "is somewhere between a physician and a nurse," I personally find that people usually grasp what you are trying to say if you describe it exactly that way.

For the technical definition of what a PA is, I will leave that up to professional organizations, such as the American Academy of Physician Assistants (the "AAPA"). According to the AAPA, the title "physician assistant" is defined as the following:

Physician assistants are health care professionals licensed (or in the case of those employed by the federal government they are credentialed), to practice medicine with physician supervision. As part of their comprehensive responsibilities, PAs conduct physical exams, diagnose and treat illnesses, order and interpret tests, counsel on preventive health care, assist in surgery, and write prescriptions. Within the physician-PA relationship, physician assistants exercise autonomy in medical decision making and provide a broad range of diagnostic and therapeutic services. A physician assistant's practice may also include education, research, and administrative services. PAs are trained in intensive education programs accredited by the Accreditation Review Commission on Education for the Physician

Assistant (ARC-PA). Because of the close working relationship the PAs have with physicians, PAs are educated in the medical model designed to complement physician training. Upon graduation, physician assistants take a national certification examination developed by the National Commission on Certification of PAs in conjunction with the National Board of Medical Examiners. To maintain their national certification, PAs must log 100 hours of continuing medical education every two years and sit for a recertification every six years. Graduation from an accredited physician assistant program and passage of the national certifying exam are required for state licensure.[1]

This may be a little long-winded for your next cocktail party. However, be prepared for this question once you share your desire to attend PA school with your close friends or family. You may be the first PA they come into contact with, and you will want to portray your new profession in the most positive light possible.

History of the profession

In my experience, it is important to know the story of how the PA profession evolved. Many, many people will ask you for more background about your profession (including some PA school interviewers). So, to address this question before you get it, I will start with a brief history of PA school. The need for physician assistants grew out of a shortage of primary care physicians. In the 1960's, physicians realized that there was a need for additional healthcare providers who could treat patients in emergency situations and in underserved areas. A physician at Duke University found a solution when he provided some ex-navy corpsmen with further training. The corpsmen were placed in a two-year experimental educational program, and when they were done, they were called physician assistants.[2]

---

[1] American Academy of Physician Assistants. Available at: http://www.aapa.org. Accessed December 20, 2007.
[2] Physician Assistant History Center. Available at: http://www.pahx.org/index.htm. Accessed on December 20, 2007.

That first program at Duke University officially began in 1965, and was limited to four students. Since then, the profession has expanded exponentially, and today there are 139 PA educational training programs, and more than 63,000 physician assistants in clinical practice.[1] With the profession in its fourth decade, you will be joining the ranks of PAs during a period of fantastic growth.

Opportunities for physician assistants

There has never been a better time to be a PA. If you pay attention to reports about "hot jobs," you will almost always see the PA profession topping the list. The United States Bureau of Labor Statistics (BLS) projects that the number of PA jobs will increase by 50 percent between 2004 and 2014. In 2006, Money Magazine reported that being a PA was one of the top 5 best jobs in America.

In addition to being an in-demand job, you probably will not be bored. PA areas of practice are extremely varied, and physician assistants can work in any specialty they want to. PAs have opportunities to work in family practice, internal medicine, surgery, cardiothoracic surgery, dermatology, ophthalmology, obstetrics and gynecology...the opportunities are practically endless! Other countries have opened their doors to the concept of PAs as well, and physician assistants that were trained in America are currently working in both primary care and military settings in England, Scotland, and Canada.

---

[1] American Academy of Physician Assistants. Available at: http://www.aapa.org. Accessed December 20, 2007.

Physician assistant scope of practice

According to the AAPA, "the scope of the physician assistant's responsibilities corresponds to the supervising physicians practice."[1] This simply means that, as a physician assistant, your scope of practice may be quite broad. In fact, that scope depends on what type of setting you work in, what the state medical boards allow, what hospital and/or clinics permit, and what your supervising physician allows.

Although the duties vary from job to job, some of the typical responsibilities PA's have include:

- Completing patient histories and physical exams ("H & P's")
- Acting as first assistant in the operating room
- Performing procedures as delineated by the supervising physician
- Providing assistance to the physician during procedures
- Evaluating, diagnosing, and treating new and existing patients' medical conditions
- Dictating patient care plans and treatment procedures
- Prescribing medications for patients (both inpatient and outpatient)
- Answering patient questions about procedures or treatment plans
- Ordering and interpreting laboratory values
- Ordering and interpreting radiology tests (x-rays, ultrasounds, CAT scans, and magnetic resonance imaging)
- Obtaining informed consent before procedures
- Documenting patient care plans and treatment procedures in each patient's chart

---

[1] American Academy of Physician Assistants. Available at: http://www.aapa.org. Accessed December 20, 2007.

In addition to the work components listed above, there is a professional practice component to physician assistant practice. After completing an accredited program and passing the national certification exam, physician assistants are expected to embody certain "moral" and "professional" characteristics. Four PA organizations (the National Commission on Certification of Physician Assistants (NCCPA), the Accreditation Review Commission for Education of the Physician Assistant (ARC-PA), the Association of Physician Assistant Programs (APAP), and the AAPA) contributed to the creation of the "Physician Assistant Competencies" which were developed to ensure that PAs enhance quality and provide accountability in health care.[1] As a PA, you will be expected to acquire and maintain the six competencies listed below:

- Medical knowledge
- Interpersonal and communication skills
- Patient care
- Professionalism
- Practice-based learning and improvement
- Systems-based practice

For a complete copy of these competencies, as well as more detailed information about them, please visit the National Commission on Certification of Physician Assistants' website at: http://www.nccpa.net.

---

[1] Accreditation Review Commission on Education for the Physician Assistant. Available at: http://www.arc-pa.org. Accessed December 20, 2007.

Why Become a Physician Assistant?

If you have purchased this book, you are obviously thinking about applying to PA school. After reading the last chapter, you have a better sense of what a PA is. With that in mind, you should next ask yourself the following questions: "Do I really want to be a PA? If so, why?" A long road follows these questions, and you must answer the first question with an honest "yes" if you are going to make it through the application process, through the education component, and then on to the challenging work you will face as a member of this profession.

Once you answer with a resounding "yes," and then decide what your motivations are, take a moment to write them down. You will need to remind yourself of these reasons when you are stressed out or overwhelmed, and you may need to use these reasons to continue to inspire you. In fact, here are some of the initial reasons I wanted to be a PA. While they are only here for illustration, you might share at least some of my ideas:

1. **Opportunities to work in the operating room.** I loved the idea of giving expert assistance to a doctor performing surgery.
2. **More opportunities for hands-on patient care.** As a dietitian, my role in the clinical setting was limited. I knew that if I became a PA, I would be able to do physical exams, participate in patient rounds, provide patient teaching, and prescribe medications.
3. **Better pay.** Before working as a PA, I was only making about $30,000 a year, and I knew that with further schooling it might be possible to double or triple that.
4. **Opportunities to help people.** Almost everyone who is drawn to healthcare wants to help people. PAs help people directly by seeing and treating patients, by providing education, and in countless other personal, hands-on ways.
5. **Interests in medicine and surgery.** I love learning, and I am fascinated by science. I wanted classes and work experiences that would allow me to better understand the human body and how it functions.

6. **Flexibility in scheduling.** Depending on the setting, physician assistants have the opportunity to work full-time, part-time, and/or per diem. This was attractive to me because I hoped wanted a profession that could provide family time, or time to pursue other academic or personal interests.
7. **Opportunities to function like a physician, without years of medical school and residency training.** Saving both time and money were both important to me, but I did not want to give up the chance to practice hands-on healthcare.

Are you sure you would not rather be a physician or a nurse practitioner?

This is probably one of the most important questions to ask yourself. You do not want to push yourself through the academic rigors of becoming a PA, and then realize you really wanted to be a medical doctor (MD), doctor of osteopathic medicine (DO), or a nurse practitioner (NP).

To help make sure you understand the role each of these professions plays in the healthcare model, as well as the educational requirements to satisfy the requirements to be one, I will take you through the current basic requirements (current as of 2008) to become a PA, MD, DO, or NP, as well as some of their basic functions in healthcare below. This will also help you to be conversant about common clinical professions if you are asked about them during your PA school interviews.

Physician Assistant

To become a PA, you must successfully complete the educational requirements of one of the accredited PA programs in the United States. PA Programs are typically 24-27 months in length, and combine both a didactic component and a clinical component. PAs are required to take and pass a certifying exam as well as obtain state licensure before they can practice. PAs are considered mid-level providers, and, under the guidance of a supervising physician, they are licensed to provide medical care autonomously in many different settings.[1]

Physician

To become a MD or a DO, you must successfully complete an undergraduate degree, as well as the educational requirements of an accredited medical school program. Medical school consists of approximately 4 years of graduate level education, and combines both didactic and clinical components. After graduating from medical school, you must apply to a residency program that provides approximately 3-7 years of additional training under the supervision of senior physician educators. Following the completion of a residency, you may decide to complete a fellowship lasting approximately 1-3 years if you want specialized training. Doctors are required to take a series of certification examinations throughout medical school, residency, and at the completion of their training. Doctors must also obtain a license to practice medicine in the state in which they work. Doctors are extensively trained because they are ultimately responsible for the treatment and management of their patients.[2]

In contrast to PAs, if a physician wanted to switch to another "field," he or she would have to complete an additional residency.

Nurse Practitioner

To become a NP, you must first complete a registered nurse training program, followed by successful completion of the educational requirements at one of the accredited NP programs in the United States. NP programs are typically 2 years in length and provide graduates with a master's degree. NPs are required to take and pass a certifying exam as well as obtaining state licensure before they can practice. NPs are considered mid-level providers, and they do not universally require physician

---

[1] American Academy of Physician Assistants. Available at: http://www.aapa.org. Accessed December 20, 2007.
[2] American Medical Association. Available at: http://www.ama-assn.org. Accessed December 20, 2007

supervision. NPs receive specialized training in one specific area of medicine for clinical practice.[1]

So, to summarize: PAs and NPs are both mid-level providers. However, NPs are limited to one area of practice (for example, family practice), but do not universally require physician supervision. In contrast, PAs can work in any type of healthcare setting (for example, surgery or family practice) but do require physician supervision. MDs or DOs are not mid-level providers; instead, they are at the very top of the healthcare-provider food chain. They take on extensive medical or surgical training so they can appropriately treat their patients, with or without the help of a mid-level provider.

Mid-level providers

The term "mid-level provider" is an umbrella title that refers to any non-physician healthcare practitioner. As a PA, you must be familiar with this term because it typically refers to both PAs and nurse practitioners. Although the original design for the roles of NPs and PAs was quite different, for both economic and healthcare access reasons, the difference between these clinicians has decreased and the scopes of practice have sometimes blended. To help you get a better understanding of the two professions, I want to review some of the similarities and differences between the two:

Similarities:

- Both PAs and NPs are considered mid-level providers.
- Both PAs and NPs can prescribe medications.
- Both PAs and NPs can work with supervising physicians.
- Both PAs and NPs as a profession have been practicing since the 1960's.
- Both PAs and NPs must pass a certification exam in order to practice.

---

[1] American Academy of Nurse Practitioners. Available at: http://www.aanp.org/Default.asp. Accessed December 20, 2007.

- Both PAs and NPs must have licenses to practice, depending on state laws.
- Both PAs and NPs are eligible for certification as Medicaid and Medicare providers.

Differences:

- PAs are trained after the "medical model" in the same manner as physicians. PA training is disease centered, with its emphasis on the biological/pathological and psychological/social aspects of health, assessment, diagnosis and treatment. Clinical training often exceeds 2000 hours.
- NPs are trained in the "nursing model," specific to nurses. NP training is biopsychosocial centered, with emphasis on health promotion, wellness, and prevention. Clinical training hours range from approximately 500-700 hours.
- PAs are dependent practitioners and are required to have a supervising physician.
- NPs are independent practitioners and can practice without supervision (depending on the state).
- PAs may have different backgrounds before becoming PAs (such as paramedics, nurses, radiology techs, medical assistants, dietitians, phlebotomists, etc…).
- NPs must first be registered nurses before becoming NPs.
- PAs can provide services in any specialty, under guidelines defined by a supervising physician, state, or hospital.
- NPs are specialized in one type of clinical practice (such as Family Medicine, Neonatology, etc…).

As you can see, there are good reasons why people sometimes confuse the two professions. In certain settings, we both provide the same services. However, as a future PA it is important that you understand the differences between the two professions, and make sure you are practicing according to the guidelines appropriate for a PA.

Are you committed enough to become a physician assistant?

Please carefully consider your commitment to becoming a PA, as attending PA school is extremely difficult and requires a significant investment of time and money. You must be completely dedicated to the program and the profession in order to successfully become a PA. This career is not for everyone; rather, this career is for people who are willing to dedicate two (or more) long years of their lives to learning all they possibly can about medicine and surgery. Remember, PAs do not need to complete a residency program like physicians. PAs get their substantive training solely during their academic program, so you must learn all you can in those two years before you are practicing on your own.

You will study. In the corridors of hospitals and medical training programs, I have heard the following comparison between PA students and medical students more than once: while the medical students have a long educational road, and sometimes take time out for "recreational activities" like playing football on campus, the PA students can always be found inside, studying. In truth, many practitioners view PA school as a condensed form of medical school, except that medical school provides a more comprehensive science and health education when compared to PA school, which typically provides students with only the necessary science and health information that students will need in order to practice medicine or surgery.

On average, **you will also spend a lot of money**, which means that you must realistically assess the cost of attending PA school. Tuition costs keep rising, and upon graduation most PA school graduates have some form of student loan debt. The average cost of PA school tuition is around $50,000 for the duration of the program. Many PA programs do not allow students to work during the programs (and for good reason). Realize that you will likely have no income during the period of time you are a PA student, because there is no free time for part-time work. If you are not willing to take on these costs, you may not be able to become a PA. Another consideration is this: if you begin a PA program, you do not want to fail or "wash out." If this happens, you will end up in the worst possible situation: you will not have the degree you paid for, and you will be stuck paying back loans regardless of your personal circumstances.

You will need the support of others. If you have a family, make sure they support your decision to attend PA school. They must understand that you will be in class almost all day long, and that you will be required to study nearly every night. They should understand that you may be working night-shifts during your clinical rotations. They must remember that you will not be able to contribute income during the time you are in PA school. If you decide to attend, make sure they are well aware of the sacrifices everyone will have to make.

Or, just make sure they read this book as well.

Reasons to reconsider becoming a physician assistant

If you have followed the steps of the book thus far, you have done a fair bit of work to consider why the profession may be right for you. However, some people want to be a PA for the wrong reasons. Hopefully, you are not one of those people. But, if you possibly are, this section may help you recognize that before you apply and become a PA student.

There are a number of reasons why I would discourage some people from becoming a PA. You might be applying to PA school as your "back-up" plan for medical school. In fact, the average PA school applicants is getting younger, because some applicants apply to PA school because they were not accepted to medical school, or because they want a safety plan in case they do not get accepted to medical school.

If you are considering applying to PA school "just in case" plan A does not work out, please save your application money. Our profession needs people who truly want to be PAs and not doctors. And, why would you want to spend all that money to become a PA only to realize 5 years down the road that you still want to go to medical school? If you want to be a doctor, apply to medical school. If you truly wish to go, there are many viable options.

If you cannot make the commitment to two or three years of dedicated study, please avoid PA school. Almost every PA program has one or two students who do not make it through to graduate from the program, and this ends up being unfortunate for everyone involved. I realize that life sometimes throws unexpected obstacles at us, but if you decide to attend a program, you must be whole-heartedly committed. Dropping out of a PA program halfway through costs you a lot of time and a lot of money, and it also keeps other deserving students from having the opportunity to enter a program. So, if you are commitment-phobic, please consider a different career path.

You should reconsider becoming a PA if you are in the profession **solely** for money or for prestige. Yes, PAs make a good living, but they work very hard. PAs also invest a lot of money into their education, which means many PAs carry significant student loan debt. As far as prestige goes, physician assistants have an important place in the medical setting. However, PAs will never have the prestige that physicians have (nor the tremendous amount of responsibility), and from my experience, most PAs do not actively seek prestige. Those that do are the distinct minority and, stick out like a sore thumb. Most PAs I have studied with or practiced with simply want to provide quality healthcare to their patients.

Finally, you should reconsider becoming a PA if you simply cannot think of anything else to do with your life. This is not the ideal postpone-your-career path or default option, and no one views PA school as the "go to law school post-BA" solution for science majors. Becoming a PA takes complete dedication to the program you are attending, and practicing as a PA requires that same dedication to our profession as a whole. As an added thought, it will be extremely difficult to do well as a student in a rigorous PA program if you really do not begin with the drive or desire to be a part of the profession.

As I have said, being a physician assistant student is difficult. I know many PAs who have said if they were asked to slog through PA school a second time, they probably would opt out because it was so difficult the first time. I admit that I sometimes feel like one of those people. That being said, there are certainly some people who had no problem balancing PA school with their outside lives; however, I have met very few of them.

The didactic, or classroom, portion of the PA program is typically the first year of the program and is usually the most difficult. Most programs require you to sit in class (and it is usually the same classroom!) anywhere from 8-12 hours per day, and then require you to study a few hours at night for a test the following morning. You generally have your weekends off, but will probably have to study on the weekends as well.

Luckily, after the didactic component, PA students reach the clinical portion of the program. Most students find the clinical portion much more enjoyable. While you will work long hours, including some overnight shifts, the clinical portion of most PA programs is much less mentally stressful because you have far fewer tests. However, the clinical portion is where students begin to feel the physical demands of being a PA. Working in the operating room (the "OR") for 12 hours, or participating in patient rounds on the floor that last 3-4 hours, will always be physically taxing on your body.

You can still have a life while you are a student, but you must prioritize your time wisely. Many students find the didactic portion of the program much more stressful, simply because it is much more mentally taxing than the clinical portion of the program. What makes the didactic portion so difficult is that you are required to learn a great deal of complex medical information in a very short period of time.

Despite all of these warnings, PA school can be quite manageable. Most students who matriculate do end up completing the program, and every school wants all of its students to graduate. However, realize at the outset what you are getting yourself into and, before it becomes overwhelming, find a way to manage the stress. Most students find some sort of outlet. Whether you choose exercise (or socializing, sleeping, watching television, journaling, etc.), the point is, if you are serious about going to PA school, you should carefully figure out your stress profile, and determine how you can manage your stress beforehand. Make a personal plan now, and then begin your PA program with your plan in mind. This is one less thing to worry about when you are too exhausted to determine your next step.

And, contrary to everything I have already told you about PA school, please do not forget to have fun while you are attending! This may be the only opportunity you have to live in a particular city, and will certainly be the last chance you will have to spend time with that particular group of students. Your fellow PA students are intelligent, dedicated people who share some of your ideals. Take advantage of this opportunity to make friends who may last a lifetime.

Aside from determining whether or not you really want to become a PA, there are other questions you must ask yourself before applying. Below, I discuss the most important considerations you should make.

Time off or straight through?

This is a difficult question to answer. Personally, I feel that those people who have taken time off after they have completed their undergraduate degree to actually gain some work experience in the healthcare field tend to have a better understanding of what working as a PA entails. If you have little or no healthcare experience, it is likely you will have little first-hand knowledge as to what a PA does and how much time and energy it takes to become one. However, if you have been working as a paramedic for two years while taking pre-requisites for PA school, you will probably have a much better idea of what a PA does.

Most admissions committees prefer that you have healthcare experience. They like to see that you have worked "in the field" and that you have decided to become a PA because you have a solid understanding of the profession. If you demonstrate this type of experience, the committees will believe that you will make a better healthcare provider because you know how physicians, PAs, nurses, and other healthcare providers work together.

Shadowing does not really provide a great deal of "hands on" healthcare experience; instead, shadowing is simply a way for you to get a glimpse of the profession. If you really want to be a PA, consider taking a year off after you complete your undergraduate degree to get substantial experience as a paramedic, nursing assistant, home health aid, or phlebotomist. Gaining actual work experience in the healthcare setting will benefit you as an applicant, and may round out your life as well. You could even find a satisfying career and decide that you no longer want to become a PA.

On the other hand, if you have been planning to become a PA since high school and have been working in healthcare throughout your undergraduate education, go ahead and apply to PA school during your last year of school. Some students actually do better straight out of college, and you may be one of those lucky few. If you feel you have all the healthcare experience you want, and you have a solid understanding of the PA profession, you are a good candidate. Just be sure to make sure to highlight those parts of your application that clearly show your dedication.

How much does physician assistant school really cost?

Simply put, school costs money. And, unfortunately, PA school costs a lot of money. For comparison's sake, and to give you your first sticker shock, I have listed the tuition numbers from several schools. Please note that this is only tuition; many schools tack on additional fees as well.

Tuition costs at various PA programs for program duration as of December, 2007:

- University of Alabama: $48,128
- Arizona School of Health Sciences: $47,350
- Loma Linda University: $63,750
- Duke University: $54,064
- Weill Medical College of Cornell University: $53,877
- Barry University: $84,000
- Central Michigan University: $46,560 (in-state), $86,280 (out-of-state)
- Midwestern University: $57,856
- Rosalind Franklin University: $41,428
- University of Iowa: $17,124 (in-state), $49,836 (out-of-state)
- Miami Dade Community College: $19,540 (in-state), $28,490 (out-of-state)
- University of California - Davis: $24,736 (in-state), $58,014 (out-of-state)
- Anne Arundel Community College: $18,861 (in-state), $38,616 (out-of-state)
- Philadelphia University: $58,506

You can find the costs for all 139 PA schools in this book's index.

These are estimates provided from the schools' websites. Of these, the average program tuition fee is approximately $43,229 which, of course, is just the beginning. You should add an additional $20,000-$30,000 for room and board, transportation and personal expenses during the program. In addition to those costs, you must add another $3,000-$4,000 for medical equipment, technology, books, and certification or licensing fees.

The total cost to attend PA school (depending on where you go) will clock in around $75,000-$100,000. If you go to an in-state program and live at home with your parents or family, your costs might be only half of that – but even then, there are no guarantees. And, either way, this is a significant investment of both time and money.

How will you pay for physician assistant school?

Most PA students (and their families) cannot afford to pay the high cost of tuition up front; however, there are several options for students who will need assistance.

Loans

The first option is student loans. There are different types of loans, and some are clearly preferable to others. A federal loan is the best type of student loan available, because the interest rate is lower than private loans. The current fixed interest rate on most federal loans as of the end of 2007 is 6.8%. There are two different types of federal loans: subsidized and unsubsidized. Subsidized loans are based on financial need, and there is no interest charge while you are in school. Unsubsidized loans are not based on financial need and do accumulate interest while you are in school. Obviously, subsidized loans are better because they are interest-free until you begin repayment. Unfortunately, you are currently limited to $20,500 in federal loans per year for tuition costs (and no more than $8,500 of that amount can be subsidized). As I show above, this is unlikely to cover all of your financial needs.

Repayment with student loans is quite flexible, and there are four different plans you can choose: the standard plan, the extended plan, the graduated plan, and the income-contingent plan. For repayment, the loans have a 6 month grace period so you do not actually have to make your first payment until you have been out of school for 6 months. If you are interested in applying for federal loans, you will need to fill out the same Free Application for Federal Student Aid (FAFSA) form you may have used in undergrad, which you can get from your school's financial aid office.

To find out more about federal student loans, you should check out the Government's website at:

http://www.ed.gov/offices/OSFAP/DirectLoan/student.html.

In addition to federal student loans, most physician assistant students will also need to take out private loans in order to cover the cost of living and any additional tuition costs. There are several different companies who provide students with private loans. Each school has arrangements with different lenders, so you may or may not have a choice in the matter. Private loans typically have higher interest rates than federal loans. The interesting thing about private loans is that you will receive the loan in the form of a personal check, and you have the responsibility to make sure it goes to the right places (rent, food, excess tuition, transportation, etc…). **Be careful!** Usually, you must make this money last for 8-12 months before you receive another check.

If you are wise, you will be good about budgeting beforehand and will only take out the amount of money (from private loans) that you will actually need. This will keep you from borrowing any "extra" money. Remember, whatever you take out, you will have to pay back with interest. Although extra money can make life a little easier while you are in PA school, it is very difficult to pay back high interest rate loans. Private loans typically have different repayment plans than federal loans. I was surprised to find out that my private loan only had one repayment option. **Make sure you have carefully reviewed your loan materials before you commit – you need to know what you are signing up for when it comes to student loans.**

Once you have been accepted to a PA program, you will be given information regarding financial aid through your PA program. In addition, the PA program should have a financial aid advisor who can help determine which payment plan is right for you.

Scholarships

Unlike undergrad, where students may attend on full-scholarship, the typical PA student gets little to nothing when it comes to tuition assistance from his or her PA program. That being said, there are several scholarships you can apply for.

If you want to go to PA school for free, your best bet is the National Health Service Corps (NHSC). Students selected as NHSC scholars receive full tuition and fee reimbursement, in addition to a monthly stipend throughout their education. The catch: the NHSC student must provide two years of service in a primary care setting that is recognized by the program as medically underserved. Before applying to this program, take a look at the list of potentially "medically underserved" areas online. Oftentimes the locations you may be assigned to are quite rural, and you will want to take this into consideration when deciding whether or not this program is appealing to you.

If you plan to participate in the NHSC program, you should apply as soon as possible. Applications are typically due in March and recipients are notified of their status in August of that year. Be forewarned, the program is very competitive. According to their website, the NHSC receives seven applications for each spot. As of now, the current website can be accessed at: http://nhsc.bhpr.hrsa.gov/index.asp

The AAPA supplies several PA students with scholarships through their Physician Assistant Foundation. As of now, the website can be accessed at: http://www.aapa.org/paf/app-scholarship.html. This application requires some essays as well as a letter of recommendation, but if you can get assistance it will, of course, be worth it.

For those potential applicants currently in the military, the Interservice Physician Assistant Program (IPAP) is a viable option. While highly competitive, the program requires no tuition fees for selected students. Following completion of this two year program, students are awarded a master's degree and are eligible to take the national certification exam for PAs. The program is located in Fort Sam Houston, Texas, and graduates receive a commission as a 1LT in the Army Medical Specialist Corps, with a post-education service commitment. Anyone serving in the military, regardless of their service, can apply for an active duty Army training seat to become eligible to participate in the IPAP program.

There are several other PA organizations that offer scholarships as well; here are just a few:

- American Association of Surgical Physician Assistants (http://www.aaspa.com/)
- Association of Physician Assistants in Cardiovascular Surgery (http://www.apacvs.org/)
- Physician Assistants in Orthopaedic Surgery (http://www.paos.org/)
- Society of Emergency Medicine Physician Assistants (http://www.sempa.org/)
- Association of Family Practice Physician Assistants (http://www.afppa.org/)
- Society of Physician Assistants in Otorhinolaryngology / Head & Neck. Surgery (http://www.entpa.org/)

Additionally, several state PA organizations offer scholarships to student members. Check with your state PA organizations to see if they offer any scholarships you can apply for.

Finally, check back in with your financial aid counselor at your PA program. He or she may know of some scholarships within the program that you can apply for.

Living on a student budget

Not only is being in PA school mentally and physically taxing, it is also financially taxing! When you are a PA student, you must learn to live on a budget. Most PA students will be living on loan money throughout the duration of the program, and may be living in a locale that is more expensive than they are used to. The average PA student must commit to living frugally.

I suggest you create a budget for yourself and stick to it. You do not want to run out of money halfway through the school year and have to apply for more private loan aid. Stick with your budget and live below your means. Pay for the essentials, such as food and transportation, but stay away from the non-essentials such as clothing and entertainment. During your clinical period, you will be likely be in scrubs anyway. I know it is tough! Trust me, I have been there, but living like a student for a few years will benefit you in the long run. Besides, your peer group of fellow students will be doing the same thing.

To help you, I have included a budget checklist on the next pages. Take the time to fill it out now, and revisit it as you prepare to begin school. A little planning at this stage of the process can save you thousands of dollars in future costs and interest payments.

Budget Checklist

Anticipated Costs	Year One	Year Two	Year Three?
Tuition			
Health Insurance			
Housing			
Food			
Transportation			
Books			
Medical Equipment			
TOTAL COSTS			

I apologize if this seems too straightforward to explain, but to estimate your total costs above, please add up the sums of Years One through Three – this will give you the approximate costs for expenses that are directly school-related. This is only a baseline for your expense – you must also include all of the extra expenses listed on the next page.

After you have worked through the entire worksheet, you will have a much better idea of what you should expect to spend on PA school. This will also arm you with information you can use when distinguishing between comparable PA schools on the basis of cost.

"Other" Fees	Year One	Year Two	Year Three?
Computer / PDA			
Certifications (BCLS, ACLS)			
Student Malpractice Insurance			
Student Disability Insurance			
Gym Membership			
TV / Cable / Phone			
Gas / Car Insurance / Maintenance			
Laboratory Fee			
University Activity Fee			
Student Health Fee			
Graduation Fee			
PANCE (exam-related fees and study materials)			
Miscellaneous			
TOTAL COSTS			

The most important part of selecting a school is your initial research. If you want to become a successful PA, you must be able to conduct research, and this is your first opportunity.

You have taken your first step by purchasing or reading this book, which will give you a foundation for beginning your search. Also, at the back of this book, I have included an index of every accredited PA program in the United States. This list should be a starting point for your search. Review the list of PA programs, highlight those you are interested in, and follow-up with even more research.

You may also want to check out the list of accredited PA programs on the AAPA website, as information frequently changes and there may be new updated contacts at some of the PA programs. The current link to the AAPA's program list website: http://www.aapa.org/pgmlist.php3. After accessing this website, view the programs you are interested in. The programs are listed in alphabetical order by state, and all of the programs' contact information is provided. Some smaller programs do not have websites listed, and I have found that occasionally a link is broken or an e-mail address is listed incorrectly. If you find this to be the case, just search for further information on the program you are interested in to find out if they have a website. Do not be shy about contacting programs – many admissions professionals are thrilled to see interest from prospective students.

Another option, for those students without time to research each program, is an on-line directory of PA programs that you can subscribe to. The Physician Assistant Education Association (PAEA) provides a website that you can purchase access to in order to find pertinent program information. The cost for this service is currently $35 per subscription. The PAEA is a reputable PA organization, and for further information visit their website at: http://www.paeaonline.org/directory/index.htm.

If you do not want to subscribe to the online directory, I would recommend you continue your research by creating a list of the programs you are interested in. Then, break down your list into subcomponents. Are you considering going out of state? Are you limited to a specific location and are you only interested in the programs near that location? Whatever your reason, decide which schools you are interested in (and I suggest you look at more than one program), and begin researching their programs.

When I began searching for PA schools, I was not limited by anything but cost, and I was open to traveling anywhere to go to school. For me, a lack of limitations made the process much more exciting because I had a huge initial number of programs to consider, and I was able to narrow it down to the top few that I thought were the best fit for me. I encourage you to first broaden your mental horizons. If you can go into the process with an open mind, you may find a program that you otherwise might have overlooked.

The best first step to learn about a program is by checking out their website. You can learn a number of things from your first visit, by asking a number of questions, such as:

- Is the website clear and easy to read?
- Is pertinent program information located on the site?
- Can I locate contact information on the website?
- Can I find out more about the faculty on the website?

If you can tell that the website has not been updated in five years, that may tell you something about the way the program operates. After checking out a program's website, you should start writing down key program information so you can compare schools. My personal advice is to make an excel spreadsheet (or write a grid out by hand) to compare each program's information. I have made a list of some of the most important items you should consider when selecting schools to apply to. I will discuss these items in greater detail following the list:

- Program Reputation
- Location
- Cost
- Type of Degree offered
- Program Curriculum

- Acceptance Rates
- Pre-requisite Requirements
- PANCE Pass Rate
- Drop-out Rates
- Housing Options
- Type of Rotations offered
- Travel Requirements during the program
- Shared Classes with other health students
- Opportunities to Study Abroad
- Opportunities to attend Advisory Sessions or Open Houses
- Opportunities to speak to former students

Reputation

You should definitely consider the school's reputation, but this should not be your only consideration. Every year, U.S. News and World Report prints an issue ranking graduate programs, and this includes PA programs. While I believe this to be a great publication, I suggest you use this guide only as part of your first consideration. Unfortunately, like most books, it has its flaws. Many schools do not participate in the U.S. News and World Report survey and are therefore excluded from the rankings. For instance, the 2006 survey only included 73 of the 139 accredited PA programs. I have no doubt that the schools listed are some of the best programs in the country, but I do believe that there are other excellent programs that were not included in the report because they did not participate. Also, pay attention to what you hear from PAs and other medical professionals. Word of mouth can help give you information about a school you otherwise may not have discovered.

Location

I think for most people location is one of the most important factors. If you have a family, you may only be able to look at a few of the programs that are closest to where you and your family are living. In fact, that is a typical reason why people apply to certain programs – simply because it is the only program close by. Do not feel bad if that is the predicament you are in; instead, consider yourself lucky to have a family support system to help get you through PA school. Your local or regional school also likely has many practicing alumni in your area, and this may help with future shadowing experiences or job searches. However, if you are like I was, and are not glued to a specific location, you should feel free to explore all types of programs to really see which one might best meet your needs.

Cost

Another important item to consider is the cost of the program. Some programs offer in-state tuition, which makes the programs much more affordable and lessens your debt load. Private institutional programs may cost much more when compared to public schools. Be honest about how much you can afford initially. If you are like most students, you will want to know how much student loan debt you will have after you have finished the program. I can personally tell you paying off student loan debt is difficult, and I guarantee most of my PA friends and colleagues feel the same way. Most PAs do have student loans and can eventually pay them off, but putting half of your salary towards your student loan payment each month is not fun. The cost associated with PA school can hang over your head for years, if not decades, so consider the cost of school carefully from the beginning.

Type of Degree Offered

Another important issue when considering programs is deciding which "degree" you want to obtain. Most PA programs have converted to master's degree programs, or are in the process of converting to a master's degree. As of now, master's degrees are the highest "PA degree" you may obtain. However, there are still many programs that only offer a certificate of completion, and others that offer a bachelor's degree or an associate's degree instead. There is no right or wrong here; all of the programs are accredited, and each will allow you to sit for the Physician Assistant National Certifying Exam (PANCE) and become an accredited PA. You should decide which degree is appropriate for you and cross off those that do not provide you with the degree you are most interested in. Just know that while the degree should not matter for clinical practice, it may affect other possible future work paths, such as teaching or pursuing other types of higher education.

Curriculum

You must consider each program's curriculum. How much time is spent on the didactic portion versus the clinical portion of the program? Which of the two are you more comfortable with? Do you personally believe you will benefit from a longer period of time in the classroom (the didactic portion) or from more time taking care of patients (the clinical portion)? Some programs are evenly balanced with 12 months of didactic training and 12 months of clinical training; however, some programs provide much more time in the classroom than on the patient floors. You should try to determine which may be better for you and better match your learning style or needs.

When looking at a program's curriculum, you should also make sure there is a cadaver lab for anatomy classes. More and more programs are getting away from the hands-on experience you get as a student in the cadaver lab, but I believe it is vital to learning the human body and to functioning as a successful PA in the future. A CD-ROM with pictures of the human body simply does not compare to the experience you get actually dissecting the human body in a cadaver lab. I speak from my own experience, and I have confirmed this with physicians and PAs I have worked with.

Acceptance Rate

Consider each school's acceptance rate. You should be able to contact the school to find out the average GPA and the total number of applicants, and you can consult my research in the index of PA programs located at the end of this book. This will help you determine whether or not the program is "within reach" for you. Obviously, if you have a 2.8 GPA and the school's acceptance average was 3.6, you may want to reconsider applying there. Or, if the school typically receives 1,000 applicants and only accepts 30 students per class, you know you are going to have to be an exceptional applicant if you are going to stand a chance at being admitted. Determine this before you apply, and you may save on application fees – as well as potential heartache if your first choice school was too far out of reach.

41

Pre-Requisite Requirements

You should determine what pre-requisite coursework is required by the PA program. If you were an English major as an undergraduate, you may have taken very few science courses. You are going to want to find a program that requires the fewest science pre-requisites because you do not want to take pre-requisites for PA school for an additional 2-3 years. However, if you were a pre-med in undergrad, this may not matter at all.

Also, keep in mind that most schools favor coursework taken at a university when compared to a community college. They also favor "upper level" science courses when compared to introductory science courses (for example, Biochem 300 is a stronger choice than Biochem 101). If you have taken all of your science courses at a community college because it was less expensive, you might be at a disadvantage. Contact the school and find out if they rank their students based on this criteria. Some schools favor the quality of the coursework, while other schools value the grade you received in the course compared to where the course was taken. This information is important because it may have a significant impact on your chances for acceptance into your chosen program.

PANCE Pass Rate

You should be able to find out the Physician Assistant National Certifying Examination (PANCE) pass rate. As I mentioned before, the PANCE is the certifying exam that PAs must take in order to become credentialed and actually practice as a PA. The "PANCE pass rate" simply refers to how many students passed the examination the first time. Many schools will advertise this on their website, but others may decline simply because their scores were low. All things being equal, if you are considering a specific school, find out that school's PANCE pass rate, especially the first-time pass rate. The rate it is indicative as to how well the school prepares their students to take the national exam and pass it, as well as how well they are training their students to practice as PAs professionally.

If I found out that many students failed the national certifying exam, I am not sure that I would want to attend that program. Your goal is to get the best quality education. Your secondary goal is then to pass the exam after you finish school. Therefore, you want to select a school that has a high

PANCE first-time pass rate. Usually, if a school has one or two students fail the exam (which is common – it is a difficult exam), the rate will still be at or above 90%. If a school's first-time pass rate is lower than that, try to find out why. The vast majority of students graduating from a well-run program should be passing the exam.

Drop-Out Rates

You should also ask how many students typically begin the program, and how many end up dropping out of the program. If there are more than one or two students that drop out each year, find out why. Is the program too difficult? Does the program allow students who may not be appropriate for PA school to attend the program simply to "get their money" before failing them out? I hope the latter is not true of any program, but if you notice a significant number of drop-outs, you should definitely be concerned as to why the program is losing students. Do not put yourself in the position to be a borderline student that may be left behind by a program.

Housing Options

If you are looking at attending a school out of state, you should find out if the school offers student housing. If available, how much will student housing cost you? If student housing is unavailable, what is the cost of an apartment in the area? Remember to include this in the budget you completed in the previous section of the book.

Types of Rotations Offered

You should find out what types of rotations are available. If you know you want to work in a particular specialty, for example, cardiothoracic surgery, find out how much time (if any) you will be able to spend participating in rotations related to your interests. Will you get elective rotations that you can choose yourself? If so, how many, and what is the duration of each rotation?

Travel Requirements

Will you be required to travel during your rotations? Some programs are set up so the didactic portion of the program is completed in its entirety at one site, and then the clinical rotations are conducted all over the state. If you are hoping to stay in one particular area because of your family, this may cause problems. In rural areas, traveling offsite (and sometimes very far offsite) is quite common. Keep potential family problems in this area to a minimum by finding out if you will be required to travel for rotations before you apply.

Shared Classes?

You should find out if the program has another graduate health program at the same site. Sometimes institutions with medical schools, physical therapy programs, and PA schools require all of those students to take some of their classes together. This is typically frowned upon because the educational programs have different learning goals, but it can and does happen at some schools. Find out if your program does this and consider whether this is something that may lessen your interest. PA school is difficult enough as is. You do not wish to be distracted, or to have program glitches lessen your interest in the curriculum.

Opportunities to Travel Abroad

Today, PA students can participate in rotations overseas during their clinical rotations. If this is something you are interested in, you should find out if the program offers opportunities like this, or other more novel approaches to teaching or clinical experiences.

Advisory Sessions

You should find out if the program has an open house or an advisory session. **If so, you should absolutely go!** These sessions are often great opportunities to meet the faculty and talk to current students. You can also tour the facilities while you are there. You should look at the classrooms and the labs. You will be spending a lot of time in these rooms as a student – do they look comfortable and well-lit, or are they dark and musty? Participating in an open house or advisory session is one of the best ways to really get a personal feel for the school and to determine whether or not it is right for you.

If you attend an open house or an advisory session, you should also send a thank you note directed to those members of the faculty who took time to answer your questions and show you around campus – so remember to get business cards or contact information at the session. If you do decide to send a note or follow-up e-mail, remember to keep it simple, professional, and to the point. Your goal is to express your gratitude and to possibly make yourself stand out just a little bit more. While some universities do not keep the letters due to space limitations, others will retain them in a file with your application.

Opportunities to Speak with Students

You should find out if there are opportunities to speak with current or former students. After connecting with a current or former student, you may learn things about the program that either discourage you, or further inspire you to attend. Current and former students of the program are some of the best resources to find out the "scoop" about the program. They will likely tell you all the good and all the bad because they are not obligated to sell the program, whereas school administrators are paid to sugar-coat their programs.

What is Missing?

After you have made your list and reviewed each school's website, find out what information is missing from the list and contact the schools directly to complete your research. These questions will elicit pertinent information that the program should be able to supply you with. I would try contacting each program via e-mail first, and if you do not get a response within a few days, then follow-up with them by phone.

Programs are used to being contacted about these issues, and most have administrative staff in place to take care of answering questions about the program. But, I do urge you to try not to be too annoying when following up with questions. You do not want to be the "annoying prospect who calls every day" with questions – that will get you the type of name recognition you do not want! Take the time to think about your questions, and write them down before contacting the program. Remember to first make sure you have explored the website and that the information is unavailable before you contact them. Call once with all of your collected questions, rather than multiple times.

The bottom line: do your research. Once you have determined which schools meet your personal preferences, you can narrow your selections down and begin the application process.

Each year, the AAPA conducts a survey to collect census information. (And, if and when you become a PA, I strongly urge you to participate in this survey as it is useful to the entire profession). If you would like to access this information, it is listed publicly on the AAPA website. As of now, you can find that information at: http://www.aapa.org/research/index.html#student.

The "average" student

I have listed the pertinent information you need to know about PA students before you apply:[1]

- The average age of PA students is 26 years old
- 72% of PA students are female
- 8% of PA students have military experience
- 29% of PA students are married
- 78% of PA students are white/Caucasian
- 48% of PA students have a bachelor's degree in biology
- 73% of PA students had worked in healthcare prior to applying (either part-time or full-time)
- 18% of PA students were Emergency Medical Technicians before PA school
- 18% of PA students were medical assistants before PA school
- 41% of PA students only applied to one PA school
- 28% of PA students applied to more than 4 schools
- 65% of PA students were accepted to one PA program
- The mean accepted PA students' GPA in undergraduate is 3.5

---

[1] American Academy of Physician Assistants. Available at: http://www.aapa.org. Accessed December 20, 2007.

- The mean amount of expected student loan debt incurred during PA school is $53,132
- 43% of PA students plan to work in family practice/internal medicine
- 36% of PA students plan to work in emergency medicine
- 32% of PA students plan to work in surgical specialties

If you are an applicant with an undergraduate degree in biology and a GPA of 3.5, with some healthcare experience, you are very likely to be accepted to PA school (and will blend in well). However, if you are a 37 year old engineer trying to apply to PA school, does that mean you will not be accepted? No, of course not. These statistics are just shown to demonstrate who the average PA student is so you can make an informed decision. Remember, not all PA students fall into the "average" category. Personally, I have no desire to be average – and I imagine that you feel the same.

Physician assistant school acceptance criteria

Every school has its own rating system as to how they select or reject students. Fortunately, some of this information is quite standard among different programs, but much of it is specific to each individual program.

Most schools have a "points" system which they use to rank their applicants, and this points system is often calculated from the information received from the Central Application Service for Physician Assistants (CASPA). CASPA is the online application program that many programs require applicants to use in order to apply to PA school. (We will talk more about using CASPA when we discuss the application process). After a school receives your information from CASPA, they typically give you a certain number of points based on the information they receive.

Most schools give you points based on:

- Overall GPA
- Natural science GPA
- Non-science GPA
- GRE score
- Any graduate credits you have earned
  (These may give you additional credits)
- Healthcare experience
- Letters of Recommendation

Some schools add or subtract additional points based on:

- Quality of education – did you attend a community college, an Ivy League school, or somewhere in between?
- Quality of healthcare experience – was it direct patient care (hands-on), or was it indirect patient care? How well did you explain or present your experience?
- Length of healthcare experience – did you work as a nursing assistant for two years, or did you shadow a PA for only two days?
- Grade trends – some schools will recognize that you may have had a bad year, but following that point your grades consistently improved. Did you explain it on your application?
- Age of academic experience – some schools prefer that coursework was completed within the 10 years of application.
- Desire to work in a specific setting – did you apply to a school that is surgically focused or dedicated to providing healthcare in medically underserved areas? If so, did you support your desire to do that type of work on your application?

The schools will also review your personal statement and will award points based on the quality of the statement. This makes it important to write a great personal statement, which is something we will talk about further in the book.

The school will calculate your total points, and if you meet a certain "minimum," you may be granted a secondary or supplemental application, or a personal interview. If you receive either of these, you should be ecstatic! It means that you have met the minimum requirements for admission, and that you will now have the opportunity to further explain why you want to attend PA school, and why you will someday make a wonderful, competent PA.

Make Yourself a Stronger Applicant

Successful applicants are able to demonstrate to admissions officers that they would be an asset to the PA program to which they are applying, and there are several things you can do as an applicant to increase your chances of gaining admission into a physician assistant educational program.

GPA

First and foremost, focus on your grades. The initial item each school reviews is your GPA, and this typically carries the most weight in the initial points calculation process. If you only have a 2.5 GPA, getting into PA school is going to be very difficult. You must improve your GPA if you want to be competitive. I know the thought of taking additional classes simply to improve your GPA may be costly, but if you are committed to being a PA, you may need to do just that. This factor may also focus your decision to even apply.

If you have a lower GPA, you should consider taking additional classes (I recommend science) or repeat courses you did poorly in. If you are simply trying to add a few classes to boost your GPA, you may want to consider taking your additional classes at a community college – it is less expensive and sometimes less intense. However, some programs frown upon community college courses, so you must take this into consideration as well.

GRE

In addition to having a good GPA, you will probably need to do well on the Graduate Record Examination (GRE). (Be sure to check whether or not your school requires you to take the GRE because not all schools do). To find out more information about the GRE, you may visit the official website at: http://www.ets.org/gre. If you have taken the GRE and done poorly on it, you should study for it and retake it. Being a PA means you will have to take multiple computerized examinations for competency in the future, so you cannot shy away from computerized exams. If you are taking the GRE for the first time, or are retaking it, I recommend that you purchase a study aid. After years of taking computerized examinations, I have found that the best way for me to learn is by doing practice exams. The study-aid agencies have books you may use to study for the GRE, as well as online and in-person programs you can purchase. To get you started, here are the most well-known study guides for the GRE:

- Kaplan (http://www.kaptest.com)
- Princeton Review (http://www.princetonreview.com)

As a baseline, I believe the minimum score you should get on the GRE for PA school is a combined 1500 in the Verbal, Quantitative, and Analytical sections, and a 4.0-5.0 on the Analytical writing section. This is a general guide – you should check with specific schools to find out what your prospective schools require.

Clinical experience

Get some clinical experience. I was personally quite lucky in that I studied dietetics in undergrad, so I was able to get substantive healthcare experience as part of my program. I realize that some people have no idea where to start. If you have a degree in English and want to be a PA, how do you get experience working in a hospital or clinic? Honestly, it is much easier than you think.

Most schools prefer that applicants have "hands-on" patient care experience. This means exactly what it sounds like: you are working in a setting that allows you to touch the patients. An example might be a nurse, or a phlebotomist. Realistically, it is quite easy to get this type of health experience – it just takes a little bit of time and money. The easiest thing you can do is to become a nursing or medical assistant. To do this, you will be required to complete a course (usually anywhere from two weeks to six months) in order to work as a certified nursing assistant (CNA), a personal care assistant (PCA), or a medical assistant (MA). The classes are worth it because you will learn skills that will be useful in your future career as a PA, and when you do get a job as a nursing assistant, you will be getting paid to hone your skills.

Another option for getting hands-on experience is becoming an emergency medical technician (EMT) or a paramedic. Again, you must complete a course in order to do this, and courses range anywhere from 6 months in length to 2 years. I truly believe that EMTs and paramedics have the best healthcare experience when they begin PA school. The EMTs and paramedics I matriculated with were extremely knowledgeable about the role of the PA and about patient care in general. They also had some of the highest grades in PA school, perhaps because of their experience. If you have the time and the money, I highly recommend this type of training.

If you are looking for a quick way to get some experience, take a phlebotomy course. Some phlebotomy courses can be taken in only one weekend. After you have received your certification, you can apply for a job in a hospital and get some experience drawing blood. Any of these paths to direct patient care will benefit you in your journey to becoming a PA.

If, for some reason, you do not have sufficient time or are unable to find a job that will allow you to get "hands-on" experience, you should still try to get non-direct patient care experience. You can do this by signing up to be a hospital volunteer, by shadowing a PA or doctor, or by working in a clinic. Also, some people in PA school had healthcare experience from work as health educators in different types of settings. There are even some former drug-reps who attend PA school. So, because the opportunities to get "healthcare" experience are as limitless as your creativity, you should be able to find something that fits into your schedule and that will benefit you as you attempt to apply to and succeed in PA school.

Shadowing experience

I mentioned shadowing in the previous paragraph. Regardless of your background, many PA schools express a preference that you have some shadowing experience before you apply. This is simply to help the schools confirm your understanding of the PA profession and the difference between a PA and a physician. If you know any PAs, ask them if they would let you shadow them. Sometimes PAs will let you shadow them for months, and other times they may only allow you to come in and follow them once. It depends on the PA and it depends on the setting. Because of the Health Insurance Portability and Accountability Act

(HIPAA) laws, some hospitals and clinics may not allow students to shadow because it "may affect patient confidentiality."

While I respect people's privacy and the law that protects that, it certainly makes getting shadowing experience more difficult. If you find a PA who says you cannot shadow them because HIPAA laws do not allow students in their organization, do not give up. You should contact other PAs or doctors to find out if they can help you find someone to shadow. You should also contact a local PA or Medical school program and ask if they know anyone who may be able to help you. And, if you still cannot find anyone, you should contact some of the professional organizations and ask them for help (for example, your state PA organization, the AAPA, AASPA, etc…).

Once you have found someone to shadow, you should take advantage of that opportunity to learn first hand what a PA does. Take notes. Ask questions about the practitioner's educational experience, their typical day at work, and their likes and dislikes about what they do. Realize that by allowing you to follow them around and by answering your questions, they are doing you a huge favor and they are taking time out of their day just for you. You should always send a thank you note afterwards. And, if you have made a good impression, you may be able to ask the PA for a recommendation letter at some point. Try to express this sooner rather than later, as you want to be fresh in their mind. A good rule of thumb for recommendation letters is to initially follow-up in one week's time, and then send a reminder two weeks later. Be professional and courteous, and you will probably get a letter of recommendation if you ask for one and are persistent in the process.

Professional organizations

Another great way to become a stronger applicant is to join a professional organization. Not only will you obtain a great deal of information about the profession by reading their newsletters or journals, but you can also network with other PAs in the organization. You will also meet other students through the organization who are going through the same process you are. In addition, you can list your membership in the organization on your CASPA application. This is just one more way you can demonstrate your interest in the profession and express your desire to become a part of it.

In the first chapter, I mentioned that I served as student director of one of the PA organizations. While I was doing this, I constantly answered questions from Pre-PA students about applying to PA school. I even spent time critiquing personal statements from students before they applied to PA school. So, do not be afraid to contact the organization if you have questions or comments. Most organizations appreciate it when people are interested in learning more about them and the profession in general.

For starters, I would recommend joining your state PA organization and/or the AAPA. If you have a specific interest in surgery, you should join the AASPA. These organizations have programs already created for "Pre-PA" students like you. Student membership is typically $50-$100. The cost may seem steep, so you should first decide if spending the money is worth it. Personally, I would say the cost is worth the opportunity to network and learn more about the profession, but I do know other physician assistants who might disagree with me. Based on your budget, decide what is best for you.

If you want to join one of these organizations, or simply want to find out more about them and read more about their activities, search for them online by the title of the organization. Here are just some of the national PA organizations:

- American Academy of Physician Assistants (AAPA)
- American Association of Surgical Physician Assistants (AASPA)
- Association of Family Practice Physician Assistants (AFPPA)
- Association of Physician Assistants in Cardiovascular Surgery (APCVS)
- Society of Emergency Medicine Physician Assistants (SEMPA)
- Association of Neurosurgical Physician Assistants (ANSPA)
- Physician Assistants in Orthopaedic Surgery (PAOS)

There are also several others you may be interested in. The AAPA has a list of the PA specialty organizations. As of now, you can access this website online at: https://members.aapa.org/extra/constituents/special-menu.cfm.

Healthcare certification courses

Another way you can make yourself a stronger applicant is by taking some relatively simple healthcare certification courses. Again, remember: whatever you can put on your CASPA application to positively present your commitment to the profession, you should. You can easily take a certification course in First Aid from the American Heart Association. You can also take a cardiopulmonary resuscitation (CPR) course as well. Go to your local American Red Cross or check out their website (http://www.redcross.org/index.html) to find out where and when the classes may be available. Earlier I mentioned taking a phlebotomy course. If you look online you can find weekend courses that provide a certification after only 2 days of coursework. If you are just looking for a quick way to get the certificate and the training, this might be the route for you.

Keep in mind that the courses above may cost as much as $400-$500 each, so you should determine how valuable you think this training might be before you spend the money. Think back, and do not forget any kind of certification you have. I know people who have listed their yoga teaching certificates on their applications, as well as their personal training certificates. Including whatever certifications you have will make you stand out and will help give the PA program a better idea of who you are and what kind of healthcare provider you might be.

Pre-PA school checklist

After reading through the information in this chapter, take careful stock in where you, as an applicant, stand today. Completing this chart will help you determine whether or not you are ready to apply to PA school. If you have marked off any items in the "no" category, you may want to consider waiting to apply to PA school until the following year so you can adequately prepare yourself.

Have you done these?	Yes	No	In Process
Taken Pre-Requisite Courses			
Shadowed a PA			
Worked or Volunteered in a Healthcare Setting			
Taken the GRE			
Made three Professional Contacts who would write Letters of Recommendation 1. 2. 3.			
Achieved a desirable GPA			
Earned Bachelor's Degree (If PA School requires)			
Decided why you want to become a PA			
Researched the Schools you want to apply to			
Created a Support Network for yourself through friends and family			
Taken a Certification Course (CPR, First Aid, etc…)			
Considered how you will pay for PA School			

How to Apply to Physician Assistant School

Applying to PA school is a life-changing decision. Once you have made the decision to apply, and believe you have completed the necessary prerequisites for admission, you then get to begin the tedious application process. And, if you thought being an actual PA student was going to be the only difficult part, welcome to the admissions process. Not surprisingly, the application process will take a great deal of work as well.

CASPA

In order to apply to most accredited PA schools, you will have to use the Central Application Service for Physician Assistants (CASPA) service. CASPA is a system that allows you to submit all of your information online in a single-application format. Once CASPA receives all of your information, it is then forwarded on to the programs to which you are applying. CASPA aims to simplify the application process, but I know many people who have had difficulty using the program.

So, to simplify the process for our own review, we must start with the basics of CASPA, the PA-specific on-line application portal. As of now, the CASPA website is: https://portal.caspaonline.org. Once you have accessed the website, you can begin the application process.

Currently, 112 of the accredited U.S. PA programs use the CASPA application system. That means that there are still an additional 27 programs that use their own proprietary applications. Before you begin entering your information into the website, check to see if your school choices use CASPA or if they use their own applications. You may need to apply online using the CASPA system for some schools, and fill out separate applications to for schools that do not use CASPA.

The most important thing I can tell you about applying to PA school is to apply early. Beat the application deadline by at least a month, if possible. The PA school application process is lengthy, and is step-by-step. If you send your application in late, you will not be considered for admission, no matter how attractive a candidate you are. The sooner the school receives your application, the sooner the school can begin evaluating you, sending you a supplemental application, and interviewing you.

You should probably create an account with CASPA as soon as you decide which schools you are going to apply to and have confirmed that at least one uses CASPA. Again, the sooner you begin, the better. Entering the information into the CASPA system is very time consuming and people oftentimes do not realize how taxing the process can be. The sooner you start entering information, the more time you get to focus on the rest of your application materials as deadlines begin to approach.

You need to be organized when using CASPA. Your first step should be to start a "CASPA folder," in which you will organize and collect all of the information you need for your application. This will include:

- Transcripts from the institutions you have attended (official copies will be sent directly to CASPA, but you may obtain student copies for your records)
- Your standardized test scores (official copies will be sent directly to CASPA, but you may obtain student copies for your own records)
- Records for any certifications you have obtained (certainly any you mention on your application)
- Your employment history
- Your health-related and/or patient contact information
- Your community service information
- Contact information for the people who will write you letters of recommendation.

Once you have collected these items, retain them in your CASPA folder. You should then create a timeline for yourself. If you know, for example, that the school of your choice has an application deadline of October 1st, plan to submit your CASPA application by September 1st. This will also help you make a timeline detailing when you will enter the necessary information into the CASPA system, as well as when you will need to order your transcripts and obtain your letters of recommendation. You need to be organized in order to finish everything related to the application process in a timely manner.

In my opinion, CASPA is fairly user friendly; however, if you are not comfortable with computers, you may have a more difficult time using the program. To begin, read the CASPA section titled, "Before Applying." Once you have done that, click on "Create a New Application." Fill in the appropriate information. The site is "secure," so you should feel safe entering personal information, such as your social security number and contact information. Write down your username and password on the inside of your CASPA folder cover so you do not forget them. You will be accessing this site frequently, so you want to make sure you can always log in properly.

Begin filling in the contact information, and carefully complete each section. Make sure you enter the information as accurately as possible. Enter all of the schools you attended, and all of the grades you received (even if some of them are not so good). **You cannot lie or exaggerate on this application – do not jeopardize your career before it even begins.** The application material will be crosschecked against your official transcripts, and you could potentially be barred from the application process if you supply inaccurate information.

While entering information on the CASPA, there are a few areas that ask you to explain your "duties." Try to keep your explanations as brief as you can. The amount of space you have to write is limited to approximately 110 words. You cannot exceed this limit because your writing will get cut off mid-sentence.

The narrative or personal statement

The narrative or personal statement is another section of the application in which the length of your writing is limited. Currently, CASPA allows for 495 words or 2970 characters, or approximately one page in Microsoft Word using Times New Roman 12 point font, single-spaced.

If you are using the CASPA system, your personal statement should "describe your motivation towards becoming a PA." And, you must describe this motivation in approximately 495 words or less. I can tell you from personal experience, limiting your personal statement to 495 words is not easy. You will have to write and edit, then re-write, and re-edit. Have several people read your essay to make sure it flows well and is grammatically correct. Read it aloud. You have less than 500 words – make sure they are perfect. Do not copy and paste it into CASPA until you are sure this is your best possible foot forward.

Before beginning your essay, take a moment to consider who you are and what you have done thus far in your life. To get you started, I have outlined a few questions you should ask yourself. Take the time to write down your answers to each of these questions – doing so may help give you ideas for your essay topic, and can help if you find yourself stuck.

- What jobs have you held, and what have you learned from each?
- What volunteer experiences have you had, and what have you learned from each?
- What healthcare experiences have you had (paid or volunteer), and what have you learned from each?
- What initially sparked your decision to become a physician assistant?
- Have you had any personal or family medical experiences that influenced your decision to become a physician assistant? If so, what were they?
- What have you learned through your shadowing experiences with PAs?
- What is unique about you? (Do you have any hobbies or talents?)
- If you applied to physician assistant school before and were rejected, what did you learn? And, what have you done since that time to improve your chances of being accepted?
- What are you currently doing to make yourself a stronger applicant?
- Have you had any unique patient experiences that have inspired you?
- Have you participated in any type of research? If so, what did you learn from it?
- Have you traveled abroad, if so what did you learn from your experience?

After answering all of these questions, you should be ready to start your essay. Simply review all of the information you have written down and see where it leads you.

I have found that the most successful personal essays are "from the heart." These essays are usually simple in nature, and tend to have a theme or a story about what inspired the applicant to become a PA. It is ok to talk about your academic history and anything unique about you (perhaps you are a concert pianist or a college athlete). You should make your essay both a reflection of who you are now and who you want to become as a PA. As with any essay, it is important to have both a strong start and finish to your essay. And, always be as clear as you possibly can. You do not need to use complicated words in your essay; you just need to write in a way that allows people to understand exactly what you are trying to say.

It is extremely important that you actually write your own essays. While you may have others help you edit your essay, make sure the material you write and submit is actually your own. Plagiarism, or any other uncredited use of another's words or ideas, are serious offenses and oftentimes have severe consequences. Many PA programs may ask you to write additional impromptu essays during your interview in order to compare the sample with your actual CASPA narrative. Please write your own essay and do not plagiarize, it simply is not worth the risk involved.

To help you get an idea of what a narrative or personal statement should look like, I have included some examples of successful essays. Each of these students was accepted to the PA program of their choice. These essays were all entered into the CASPA system, and each is less than 2970 characters. Decide which ones you like and do not, but remember that these were all "winning essays," such that the students who wrote them were accepted to a PA program. Pick one, or several, whose style seems comfortable, and try writing your first draft with that style in mind. Remember, use these essays to generate your own ideas, not to copy other individuals' material.

Essay One:

Working as a certified Pilates Instructor, I have been fortunate to have the opportunity to assist numerous people of varying fitness levels and abilities. Pilates balances my two passions: biology and contemporary dance – each an undergraduate major. My experience with and admiration for a particular client, a woman named Kirby, helped me to appreciate the limitations of a Pilates Instructor and reinforced my desire to become a healthcare professional. Kirby and I worked jointly in setting fitness goals out of her desire to alleviate discomfort from osteopenia by strengthening core and back muscles and to improve her golf game by increasing flexibility. After devotedly working twice each week for several months (she worked more diligently than many of my clients half her age) there was visible improvement in Kirby's core strength to the extent that I often forgot she was in her late seventies. One Wednesday, shortly following our weekly training session and while out playing her customary round of golf, Kirby, tragically and suddenly, expired on the course. Shocked and saddened, I consequently became aware that while I had had the capacity to improve Kirby's fitness level and outward body conditioning, an internal ailment, one undetected and untreatable by any amount of Pilates training, ultimately caused her death. It became clear to me that it would be tremendously rewarding to be informed and involved on yet another level, one that would require further training and additional skills.

Earlier, in the process of completing a research technician internship at Johns Hopkins University Institute of Genetic Medicine during the summer following my junior year, I had felt the stirrings of a desire to combine my love for the health sciences with a career that involved human interaction. While fully aware that I was at least indirectly contributing toward the greater understanding of genetic disorders through my research efforts, I much preferred the observation of and personal contact with young patients with various disorders during my days at the hospital's genetic clinic. My internship left an indelible appreciation for medical research, but the satisfaction I received from interaction with those children had begun to show me that my personality is better suited for the types of mutually rewarding relationships that can be established between Physicians Assistant (PA) and patient.

The process of working with clients one to three days each week in private Pilates training sessions has provided invaluable experience toward becoming comfortable in working with people on an intimate level. It has been a privilege to share in a client's recovery or to help them to achieve their fitness goals. Through my shadowing experiences with several PAs, I have gained insight into the daily regimen and requirements of the profession. The opportunity to observe PA interaction with doctors and nurses within the operating room environment has further reinforced my belief that a career as a PA is the proper fit for my personal and professional goals within the medical field. I feel confident that both my education and professional experience have prepared me for this rigorous, rewarding and most exciting next step.

Essay Two:

I am extremely motivated to pursue a challenging career as a physician assistant because I enjoy mental stimulation, the chance to increase my knowledge, the expanded scope of practice, the increased involvement with my patients, and providing access to quality healthcare that is more affordable.

Currently as a paramedic, I encounter a variety of cases that seem similar on the surface, but are each quite different. I enjoy this puzzle-solving aspect of my job. As a PA, increasing my scope of practice and depth of treatment will provide the mental challenges I need to be fulfilled in my career.

To achieve my goal of gaining new knowledge and understanding, I have attended many classes and seminars that have given me a broad base to draw from so that I can treat my patients more skillfully. The higher level education of PA school will greatly increase my knowledge and provide flexibility to choose from many different and challenging specialties and sub-specialties.

I also wish to develop deeper relationships with my patients. As a paramedic, I only see my patients for the time it takes to get to the hospital. As a PA, I will be able to interact with my patient in more than one encounter which will assist me in providing a higher level of care by developing a rapport. That deeper relationship will help me to know my patient: a patient needing cardiac rehabilitation for example, who is the primary caregiver for her husband whom has Alzheimer's disease and feels that she has already spent too much time away from her husband, and to use that knowledge to devise the most appropriate treatment plan that my patient will be compliant with.

I am also concerned with the growing costs of healthcare and the ability to access quality healthcare. By becoming a PA, I know that I will be out on the frontlines, providing quality, more affordable healthcare, as part of a MD/PA care team. I know that Americans today, along with institutions such as Medicare, Medicaid, and HMOs recognize the ability of a PA to provide quality healthcare which is more affordable.

I know that by becoming a PA, I can be a part of the solution to our current and future healthcare crises, knowing that as a part of an involved healthcare team, our patients will benefit from our efforts.

Essay Three:

After pioneering a special education camp in my hometown for underprivileged, handicapped children and helping care for a young boy with Muscular Dystrophy during my high school years, I felt compelled to continue activities such as these during my collegiate career. With this driving force behind me, I chose to get involved in two research projects. The first project examined the locomotor activity in infants with Spina Bifida while the second project analyzed gait patterns in infants with Down Syndrome. Since both illnesses lead to irregular walking patterns, we sought to find interventions that would grant these infants the ability to walk during the same timeframe as children who develop normally. Although this study was often disheartening, from the child that would not participate in the data collection if I was not present to the young boy who struggled with each step, the remarkable progressions of each child gave me renewed energy. Even if these children were afflicted with life-altering disabilities, I realized that encouragement played a vital role in their walking improvement and general self-confidence. The role of the child's family and other workers had clear implications on the child's drive to succeed.

While engaging in these research projects, I worked and volunteered in hospitals and nursing homes. I was often inspired and gratified to hear of a patient's encounters with empathetic nurses and comforting friends and family; I was again reminded of the importance of social support and encouraging words. To further my understanding of individuals who overcame their illnesses with a strong supportive network and hardy mind, I was motivated to write an honors thesis on social problem solving. Through this research, I found that improvements in health, as well as regressions in health, were in direct correlation with the amount of social support surrounding the individual. This in turn helps form their problem solving skills and can have astounding effects on their illness-coping abilities. My thesis is now in review for publication. Since then, I am now the editor of a book titled, "Mental Health in Medical Settings: A Multidisciplinary Approach." With collaboration from reputable clinicians, this book describes the role of mental health in medical settings from the viewpoints of professionals such as psychiatrists, nurses and social workers. Our goal is for the publication to provide helpful insights into the interaction between mental and physical health.

As I branch into the next chapter of my life in pursuit of a career as a physician assistant, I am eager to incorporate these experiences into the care of my patients, since they have indeed molded my motivation for becoming a PA. Through the numerous areas in which I have researched the impacts of supportive networks and self-assured care, I hope to better serve the needs of my patients on both psychological and physical levels.

Essay Four:

Throughout my pursuit to excel in academia, I have also maintained and enhanced my professional career. The skills and knowledge I acquired from my work experience aided me in my biomedical science curriculum and also strengthened my interest in the clinical sciences. Initially during my undergraduate studies, I had applied for local volunteer positions; fortunately, I was hired instead as a research assistant for Yale University. The experience of working as a research assistant presented me with a myriad of opportunities, such as working directly with patients, participating in a student fellowship, and presenting at a national conference. A few of my clinical responsibilities included monitoring patient behavior, collecting vital statistics, conducting various cognitive and physical tests, and maintaining communication with medical staff.

After graduation in May of 2003, I began working for the Centering Pregnancy Program at Yale University. The main focus of the study was to reduce the risk of HIV and other STDs during and after pregnancy among ethnically diverse young women receiving prenatal care in public clinics. My clinical responsibilities included working with medical staff during pre-natal care provided to our patients and maintaining communication regarding the health of our patients during their pregnancy. I enjoyed working in the clinic and I was fortunate to have been exposed to an integral aspect of public health. I went on to working for Advanced Endodontics as a dental assistant and my clinical responsibilities included interacting with patients and assisting the doctor during endodontic procedures including surgery.

While employed by Advanced Endodontics, I realized I wanted to further my studies and enrolled in the Master's in Medical Laboratory Sciences program, which I successfully completed this spring (2006). During the second year of my Master's, I applied to neuroscience PhD programs; however, I realized that although I enjoyed the research aspect of the studies I have worked with professionally and academically, I found each to be rewarding more so because of the opportunities I had to interact with patients in the clinical setting.

With the new 80-hour workweek being implemented in residency programs and the increasing demands for qualified Physician Assistants, I looked into the Physician Assistant field and developed a keen interest. I turned down an acceptance from the University of Connecticut for their Neuroscience PhD program in order to pursue my growing interest in the Physician Assistant program. I also had the opportunity to shadow a PA at Yale New Haven Hospital and found her knowledge of the clinical health sciences and her skills in providing care for her patients to be truly inspiring.

Based on my experiences thus far, I would like to expand my knowledge of the clinical health sciences and increase my exposure to patient care by enrolling in the Physician Assistant Program.

Essay Five:

Once, not long ago I was his surgical patient; now, I was standing inches from that surgeon as he made his final incisions to excise the invading cancer. Having experienced emergency surgery myself, I know first hand how significantly a physician can touch someone's life. Simply put, he saved mine. And, by observing his work on this procedure, I watched the surgeon prolong yet another patient's life. These experiences, combined with the opportunity to help each patient and to perhaps tackle a new challenge with each and every case, help define my desire to pursue a career as a physician assistant.

Since childhood I have had an interest in the medical field. Early scholastic dissections captivated my interest on how the human body functions, and I became enthralled by the interaction of organs and bodily chemical reactions. However, disappointments and setbacks have sometimes affected my goals and dreams. In particular, when I was a student at Wells College, I struggled with illness and emotional distractions and became extremely unhappy. This combination of stressors, consequently, was reflected in my grades. I decided to make a dramatic change, and transferring to the College of Mount Saint Vincent proved to be a very positive decision for me. In order to graduate on time, I did have to increase my workload; nonetheless, rising to this challenge was extremely fulfilling and I made the most of my new opportunity.

As a current team member with the Young Adult Institute/National Institute for People with Disabilities, I work with eight individuals on a daily basis. I have witnessed "Lucy," a client diagnosed with mild mental retardation and epilepsy, suffer through many grand mal seizures. Each seizure reminds me of my desire to help her more. Although I understand there are positive as well as negative considerations to any surgery, my heart goes out to Lucy because I feel that she is being denied the opportunity for a better quality of life. As a candidate for epilepsy surgery, she has the chance to live a nearly seizure-free life. Her legal guardian, however, vehemently opposes this option; subsequently, Lucy must endure a severely impaired existence. While I have limited influence on this aspect of her life, I long to be a member of the team performing successful surgeries and helping patients like Lucy.

I remain committed to working with each of my clients by advocating, counseling, and assisting them medically. However, I wish to do more. My experiences as a patient, intern, and employee have exposed me to the medical field from many different perspectives, and through each experience, I have continued to search for new avenues to help people. My desire to pursue a career as a physician assistant, where I can dynamically help as well as learn new and innovative medical techniques, has grown from those experiences, and has led me to apply to PA school.

Essay Six:

What strikes me most about the operating room is the dialogue that takes place between the physician assistant and the surgeon. Both moves in tandem, seamlessly, with senses keen to the needs of the patient. On one occasion, I can recall watching the surgeon's precise and exact movement, and the physician assistant's agility in responding to the procedures complexities. As the physician assistant closed the incision, my passion for becoming a surgical physician assistant ignited.

While the past five years of my life have been educationally dedicated to enhancing my knowledge in the areas of nutrition, disease, and wellness, I have always taken an active interest in health. From competing for the Presidents fitness test in elementary school to performing animal dissections by high school, health has remained a passion. My role as a dietitian has given me a variety of experiences in clinical and community settings. On the clinical side, I have utilized biochemical data, functional status, and pathophysiological conditions to identify appropriate nutritional needs of patients. I have developed and modified care plans for a diverse patient population, including consultations for those that receive nutrition support. In the community setting, I have lead nutrition classes and provided nutrition-related home visits to those in medically-underserved populations.

Initially attracted to the physician assistant profession by the opportunity to play a bigger role in patient care, my experience shadowing physician assistants has reinforced my decision to pursue the career. Through shadowing physician assistants in the clinical setting, I have been able to see the impressive results of disease-specific patient care. Similarly, spending time with a physician assistant in a community clinic helped me fully grasp the necessity of a wide range of medical knowledge that the expansive medical needs of patients require. I look forward to using these insights, along with future shadowing exercises, in my path to becoming a physician assistant.

My enthusiasm to enter physician assistant school drives me to pursue new challenges; I am currently taking additional health science classes to better prepare myself for the intense curriculum of the physician assistant program. I have recently become certified in phlebotomy to develop skills in venipuncture and aseptic techniques. As a member of the AAPA and the AASPA, I am learning more about current trends in the profession. As evidenced by my professional experiences and current pursuits, I am preparing myself to play a larger role in patient care by becoming a physician assistant. This broad range of involvements, coupled with my dedication and enthusiasm, have given me and excellent foundation of which to begin this endeavor. I am confident that as a physician assistant student I will bring an energetic attitude and an unparalleled vigor for learning, both in and out of the classroom.

Essay Seven:

Since the beginning of my journey as a college student, I have overcome many obstacles in reaching a decision regarding my future career. One thing that remained constant was how I could not see myself anywhere other than the medical field. Even though I felt unsure, I kept taking the required classes. One night, at an AED Pre-Health Honor Society meeting, we had a speaker who was a second year student from the University of Alabama in Birmingham's Physician Assistant Program. I did not know much about this profession; however, everything the speaker described seemed to fit my exact career goal characteristics. After the meeting, I was so intrigued that I stayed and talked to her for almost two hours. That was the moment I knew that I wanted to become a Physician Assistant. Since that night, I have found myself searching for hours at a time on the internet about facts, organizations, and recent journal articles about this intriguing field of medicine. I have joined the American Academy of Physician Assistants, from which I receive up-to-date articles about this growing profession. This fall I am taking a shadowing course, and following graduation in December, I plan to intern at a local hospital, hopefully in surgery. I have grown more fascinated with surgery after observing various heart procedures and seeing how much autonomous work a PA does. According to the AASPA, the surgical PA really is "the best instrument a surgeon has."

In my opinion, the most important role of a Physician Assistant is to be there for the patient before, during, and after their hospitalization. I want to know my patients on a personal level that stems from their daily routines, such as Mrs. Jones' love for gardening and how she has trouble enjoying it due to carpal tunnel syndrome. If I can help people do everyday things that they love, I will have fulfilled my goal as a person and a health care provider. I have learned that one of the places in a hospital where patients can be treated impersonally, many times unaware by the staff, is in surgery. This is actually the place where the majority of patients need the most emotional guidance and comfort. Many are fearful and uncomfortable about going under the knife and all they want is to hear an encouraging voice to lighten their anxiety. I, as a PA, want to be that person that calms a little girl's fear of getting her tonsils removed, pray with an older man battling cancer, or congratulate a woman on the birth of her baby. Another important factor in being a PA is communicating. I have been sick in another country and being able to communicate with the doctors was very helpful. I want to be able to understand a patient, whether it is in Spanish or Sign Language. I feel that Physician Assistants have a passion that is sent out to the people that need it most. I want to be a part of this team; therefore, I would greatly appreciate your consideration for a place in the next class.

Entering your academic history

If you are using CASPA, entering your academic history will probably be the most difficult and tedious part of the process. First, you must enter each institution you attended, followed by each class you took, which term it was taken during, and your grade. This means you must have copies of your transcripts in front of you while you are entering this information. You do not want to enter any information incorrectly, so be sure to double check everything.

In addition to entering all of your grades, you must also send CASPA an official copy of your transcript. You must print out the transcript request form (from the CASPA website) and send it to each institution you attended. Some institutions charge a fee for your transcripts, and others do not. I would advise you to begin this process early so you can monitor, via the CASPA website, whether or not your transcripts have been received.

Check to make sure the information below is current, but as of now, you should send your official transcripts to the following address:

CASPA
Transcript Department
P.O. Box 9108
Watertown, MA 02471

Another part of the academic history portion of CASPA is entering your standardized test information. According to the CASPA website, if you have not taken the GRE yet and your school requests it, you should designate that the GRE scores be sent to that particular school when you take the exam. However, if you have already taken the GRE, you can simply enter in your scores into the CASPA website and they will verify that information based on your social security number. If you are entering information about other standardized exams (TOEFL, AP coursework, etc…), please refer to the CASPA website.

Letters of recommendation

Obtaining letters of recommendation can range anywhere from fun to excruciatingly painful, but here are my suggestions to make the process as painless as possible: first of all, you need to decide who to ask. As of now, CASPA requires three letters of recommendation. Find out if the institutions you are applying to have any requirements as to who the letters are written by. Some PA programs require the letters be written by physicians or physician assistants, while others have no requirements. You can have the person you choose either enter their letter electronically through a secure website, or via paper form, where they write the letter and send it into CASPA. Ask the person who will be writing the letter for you which way they would prefer to do it.

You should understand that letters of recommendation do not weigh extremely heavily in the scoring process when compared to grades and healthcare experience. That being said, a letter of recommendation that is not favorable can still hurt you in the application process.

I know a person who applied to graduate school after attending a major university. In a very difficult chemistry class with nearly 400 students, she was one of 10 students to receive a 4.0 grade. She decided to ask the professor of that class to write her a recommendation letter because she thought that since she did so well in the class, he would think highly of her and write a great letter. She was wrong! The professor did write a letter for her, but unfortunately the letter said very little that was positive about the student. The professor commended her for getting a good grade in his class, of course, but also said that he did not know her because the class was so large, and he had never worked with her one-on-one.

Learn from her mistake. When deciding who to ask for a recommendation letter, you should choose someone that knows you very well. The strongest letters of recommendation will come from professors, PAs, MDs, DOs, or even nurses who know you well, who can verify that you have the drive to become a great physician assistant, and can state that you will succeed in a rigorous academic environment. If you shadowed a PA or physician, you may want to ask them for a letter. You should also have a professor write you a letter of recommendation. Make sure the professor you choose is someone who can comment on you favorably as a person, and not just state that you did well in his or her class.

Remember, it is your responsibility to get to know your professors, and to get to know a professional who will write you a strong letter of recommendation. You simply must make this effort when you have the opportunity. Keep an address and contact information on file for each professional contact you meet. You will need them for CASPA.

When using CASPA for the electronic version of the letter of recommendation, you need to enter in all of the letter writer's personal information. CASPA will then send that person an "electronic request" asking them to fill out your letter on their secured website. You should follow-up with your letter writer to make sure they received the "electronic request" and to make sure they completed the letter of recommendation.

One nice thing about the CASPA system is that you can check the "status" of your letters of recommendation and transcripts to find out if they have been received, or if they are still pending. Therefore, once you have asked people to write letters of recommendation for you, be it in electronic or paper form, it is your responsibility to monitor the status of your letters and to make sure those people you have asked complete them in a timely manner.

If you have asked someone to write a letter of recommendation for you, please send them a thank you note afterward. Writing a recommendation letter is very time consuming, so you should thank those who wrote letters for you for the time they took out of their already busy schedules. And remember, you may need their help in the future as well.

Supplemental applications

Some schools require you to complete a supplemental application in addition to submitting your materials to CASPA. While the CASPA website specifies whether or not you need to submit a supplemental application, I urge you to contact your specific school(s) to verify this information. Some schools request that your supplemental application be submitted at the same time as your CASPA application, while others do not send you a supplemental application unless you meet the minimum requirements for admission into their program. Many schools provide information regarding supplemental or secondary applications on their website. I have also included this information in the index of PA pro-grams at the end of the book.

Don't forget: A few things to remember about CASPA

Using the CASPA system does cost money. And, unfortunately, the more schools you apply to, the more money it costs. As of now, the current cost for CASPA starts at $160 for one school and adds an additional $30-$40 for each additional school you apply to. So, if you apply to four schools through CASPA, it will likely cost you $270. Budget for this amount from the beginning, but you will not pay CASPA's fee until you actually click "submit" and send all of your information to CASPA.

Remember to send these items via U.S. Mail to CASPA:

- Letters of Recommendation – either electronically or paper form
- Transcripts – make sure you order and send official copies

If you have problems with CASPA, do not hesitate to call them. I spoke with them when I had problems during my application, and they were quite helpful. As of now, you can reach CASPA at:

Telephone: 617-612-2080
E-Mail: CaspaInfo@caspaonline.org

On the next page, you will find a checklist that should help you organize the materials you will need to successfully complete the CASPA process.

CASPA Checklist

Completing this chart will help you determine whether or not you are ready to "E-submit" your CASPA application. Once you have completed all of the items on the checklist, you should feel confident that you are ready to send your application on for admissions review.

Have I completed the following?	*YES*
Ordered my Transcripts	
Selected three people to write Letters of Recommendation and sent those people the CASPA Information **1.** **2.** **3.**	
Sent in my Supplemental Applications (If your schools require these)	
Carefully entered my GRE Information (If required to)	
Carefully entered my Contact Information	
Carefully entered the Institutions I attended	
Carefully entered my Health Related Training	
Read my Personal Statement out loud	
Had friends and family read and review my Personal Statement	
Carefully Spell-Checked and Grammar-Checked my Personal Statement	
Carefully entered my Narrative or Personal Statement	
Carefully entered my Health Related Experience	
Carefully entered the Programs I want CASPA to send my Information to	
Carefully entered my Personal Data	
Carefully entered my Coursework	
Carefully entered any Additional Information	
Carefully entered my Patient Contact Experience	
Carefully entered my Other Employment	
Carefully entered my Community Service Experiences	
Double Checked all of the Above!	

Secondary Applications

If you receive a secondary or supplemental application (the two are interchangeable), you have successfully made the first cut. Congratulations! However, you are not done yet. In order to make it through this next step, you will want to follow the directions on the secondary applications carefully.

Typically, when programs send out secondary applications, they are trying to get a better sense of your depth of knowledge regarding healthcare in general, and specifically the PA profession. The typical secondary application consists of a number of essay questions that you must answer.

If you receive a secondary application, the first thing you should do is read the directions very carefully. Second, you should make several copies of the application. Some applications require handwritten essays, so, if you find that you need to handwrite your answers, you will want to avoid using the original copy the first time you write it out. Just imagine – you have written out your essay on the original application, and realize, with ten words to go, that your essay, written lovingly in black ink, is so long it does not fit on the page. That has certainly happened to students before. Make sure it does not happen to you!

To start answering the questions, you should first do some research. A lot of the questions are typically related to PA reimbursement, the role of the PA in comparison to the NP or the physician, and some may even be a bit more personal – asking you to explain a personal story about your healthcare experience. Whatever the questions are, make sure you do the appropriate research. You can use whatever resources you need to – make sure you have read through this book in its entirety, talk to people, read articles on the internet, and look to PA organizations. I also encourage you to have several people read your essays to make sure they are grammatically correct and that they make sense.

When you have perfected your answers, practice writing them on the copies you made to confirm that they fit. Once each fits, write them on the original copies and make sure you write it in your best handwriting. I cannot tell you how many secondary applications I have seen where the handwriting is hardly even legible. When I am scoring essays and I see the applicant has not taken the time write legibly, while I try to remain unbiased, I am probably more inclined to score the essay poorly. I emphasize again, write the essays in your best handwriting, or ask (or pay) someone with nice handwriting to transcribe it for you.

Finally, pay attention to the deadline. Secondary applications are usually due within 2 weeks of receiving them. Make sure you send them out before the deadline so they arrive on time. If you are concerned about the PA program not receiving the secondary, you can always call the program, or send an e-mail to check. Back up your records by sending the application via certified US mail or an overnight service with package tracking.

When I applied to PA school, only one school provided its applicants with secondary applications. Nowadays, secondary applications are used much more frequently. In order to give you an idea of what a secondary application may be like, I am listing some typical questions, followed by actual PA student answers. Again, please use these only as guides.

1. Explain why you want to become a PA.

> With a registered nurse as a mother, I was introduced to the healthcare field at an early age. Although I admired my mother's career choice, I felt compelled to pursue a different path. While I was working as a dietitian, I was exposed to the role of the physician assistant and through my desire to play a larger role in patient care; I became interested in the profession.

> I have tremendous respect for physicians, but I have never wanted to pursue this career for myself. I feel my time would be better utilized as a physician assistant, allowing me to provide patient care at a similar level in a shorter period of time. Although physician assistants are not trained in the exact manner as physicians, I believe using the medical model is highly advantageous for it allows greater opportunity to work in varying specialties. Unlike physicians or nurse practitioners, I like the fact that physician assistants are dependent practitioners with the ability to work

autonomously. Because of this integrated care system, physician assistant's work in complementary and synergistic ways with physicians, providing exemplary patient care.

2. *Explain an unforgettable healthcare experience you have had.*

While working in an outpatient clinic, Megan, a newly diagnosed juvenile diabetic patient came in for diet counseling with her parents. I could sense she was frustrated and confused about counting carbohydrates and checking her blood glucose levels daily. My heart went out to her as she struggled to comprehend this genuinely overwhelming amount of information. After a two-hour consultation, I was sure we had made some progress. I quizzed her by giving her some sample portion sizes of a few foods, and (to our delight!) she was able to identify the correct carbohydrate exchange. I witnessed the excitement in the patient's newly enlightened eyes as she understood why diet is important. Megan returned to the clinic every few weeks for follow-up visits and her progress was remarkable. Her blood glucose legs revealed she was controlling her diabetes extremely well, an amazing feat for an eight- year old girl previously terrified to poke herself in the finger. This experience helped me realize my passion for working with people and making a difference in their lives.

3. Explain managed care to the best of your understanding.

Managed care plays a significant role in how healthcare providers are able to treat patients. In some ways it seems as though insurance companies have the ability to determine the type of care patients may receive. For example, each patient is only allowed to stay in the hospital a specific number of days based on the patient's diagnosis. Because managed care provides just enough treatment to correct the patient's current problem, the shortened length of stay will continue to be a dilemma. This will probably require physician assistant to treat more patients, ultimately curtailing the time they are able to spend with each patient. Managed care also dictates what medications patients may receive, which can make treating a patient more difficult for healthcare providers, such as physician assistants. Unfortunately, these changes may have a real and significant effect on the quality of care physician assistant provide. While managed care appears to have temporarily slowed the rapid increase in health care costs, I am curious as to how the healthcare system will evolve as the cost of healthcare continues to rise.

4. Differentiate between SARS and AIDS.

SARS, the latest global killer spreading like wildfire, mimics the AIDS outbreak of the early 1970's. A key reason SARS and AIDS have been compared to each other is the high number of people infected in such a short period of time. The SARS outbreak has infected more than 8,400 people around the globe proving fatal for at least 800 people in less than six months, while AIDS has infected more than 42 million people worldwide and has claimed an estimated 25 million lives. AIDS has resisted development of a vaccine by mutating rapidly and SARS has already demonstrated a similar capability.

One major difference between SARS and AIDS lies in the containment strategy. With AIDS, it took years to classify the disease, determine the source, and define the populations at risk. With SARS, researchers were able to determine these factors within a few short months and quickly put preventative and isolation measures into place. AIDS requires fluid contact between people for transmission and is a preventable, behavior-related disease. SARS, however, is airborne and can exist on surfaces such as doorknobs and elevator buttons for hours – making it nearly impossible to prevent. The outbreak of SARS underscores our vulnerability to new infectious diseases. Although SARS spread quickly, the rapid international response mitigated the damaging effects of the disease.

5. Explain why you think the PA profession is growing.

There are several reasons for the growing PA profession. First, because of the increased number of patients that a physician needs to see on a daily basis in order to be economically compensated, PAs multiply the number of patients seen. Thus, it is necessary for physicians to employ PAs in an attempt to extend their care and serve a greater number of patients. Secondly, with the restricted number of hours that a resident may work, these hours are now being overturned to PAs. Thirdly, with the increase need to specialize on the part of physicians, PAs have become the generalist for many aspects of the patient's primary care. Lastly, the healthcare industry as a whole is expected to experience a greater need for healthcare professionals as a large percentage of the population ages and retires.

Physician Assistant School Interviews

So, you have been granted an interview. Congratulations again! Now that you have the opportunity to show the school who you are in person, you should make the most of it. Interviews can be quite different from school to school. Some schools interview as many as 50 students all on one day, while others only interview three or four students at one time. The typical interview day begins with a "welcome" session where potential students are introduced to some of the faculty members and given a tour of the school. Sometimes they are asked to participate in a quick writing test. Be prepared: do not party late the night before, since schools use this test to assess your ability to think and write clearly in a short amount of time. After the test, candidates are then given a tour of the school and some of the classrooms. Finally, students are typically interviewed by a few different members of the faculty and, in some cases, by students currently enrolled in the program.

In order to fully prepare for the interview, you need to do some research first. You will need to learn about the PA program you are interviewing at, as well as more about the profession in general. Print out information about your school beforehand, and bring it with you for reference. You will also need to practice answering some sample interview questions out loud. Have a family member or friend ask you practice questions so you can get used to answering them. By answering the questions out loud, you may realize that you do not really know what you are talking about. I suggest you research the following questions. You may or may not be asked these questions, but it never hurts to be prepared.

Topics you should be comfortable talking about should include:

- The role of the PA in healthcare
- The difference between PAs, NPs, and MDs or DOs
- How PAs are reimbursed
- Different practice settings PAs can practice in
- Why you want to be a PA
- Why the PA program should choose you
- How you will deal with the stress of the program
- What type of work you want to do as a PA (Family practice, plastic surgery, etc…)
- Why you are interested in this specific PA program
- How you are unique from other PA candidates the school is interviewing
- What are your own strengths and weaknesses?
- What are your hobbies?
- Do you work well with others, or do you prefer to work by yourself?
- How does your family feel about you going to PA school?
- What will you do if you are not accepted to PA school?
- What do you imagine PA school will be like?
- What do you imagine PA practice will be like?

Some programs like to throw in random questions to see how you will respond. If you are asked a silly question, such as, "If you were an animal, what animal would you choose to be?" just answer the question as creatively and quickly as you can. Do not worry – they simply want to see if you can think on your feet.

You may also get asked questions that relate to current trends in healthcare or scenarios that you might find yourself in as a PA. It is hard to prepare for these types of questions. I recommend doing your research to make sure you have a basic understanding of the current laws related to PA reimbursement, and Medicare/Medicaid. And, of course, you have read this book, which provides many of the basic ideas concerning PA practice. As for health scenarios, I can give you an example:

> You are the PA working in the Emergency Room and you are evaluating a 14 year old girl who presented with abdominal pain. After examining her, your nurse informs you that the urine sample you ordered earlier shows a very high level of Beta hCG indicating that your patient is likely pregnant. What do you do?

Questions like these are difficult to answer, and if you are given one similar to this, just try to answer it the best you can. If you do not understand something, it is ok for you to say, "I don't know," or, "I am not sure." Remember, you are not a PA yet, so you should not be expected to know everything that a PA would know already. By giving you questions like these, interviewers are just trying to assess your ability to think critically and to give sound, reasonable answers. If you are unsure of the answer they are looking for, explain that under these circumstances, you would look up the answer in order to make sure you could correctly diagnose and treat the patient.

As with any interview, you should always be prepared to ask some questions of your own. Here are some questions you should remember to ask:

- Why should I choose your program?
- What is a typical day like during the didactic portion?
- What is a typical day like during the clinical portion?
- Are there any special programs for which this PA school is noted?
- How well do your students typically do on the PANCE exam?
- Has this PA school ever been on probation or had its accreditation revoked?
- How are students evaluated academically?
- Is there a mechanism in place for students to evaluate their professors and attending physicians?
- Are there any scholarships within the program I can apply for?
- What kind of academic and personal counseling opportunities are available to students?
- Are there computer facilities available to students?
- Are computers integrated into the curriculum or learning activities?
- What type of learning modalities does the program utilize? (Problem-based learning, lecture, hands-on, etc…)
- Before I begin the program, are there any additional courses or work experiences I should try to take advantage of?
- How long does it take for most graduates of your program to find jobs?
- What type of preparation do you provide your students with before taking the PANCE exam?
- Is a car necessary for clinical rotations? If so, are parking passes provided?
- Are students involved in community service?
- Are there any opportunities for rotations abroad?
- Does the school have a cadaver lab? If not, how is anatomy taught?
- Will I be taking classes with other medical students or physical therapy students, or is the program completely separate?

Take notes! If you attend a number of student interviews, at the end, you may not be able to differentiate between schools. Good note-taking will help remind you of each school's strengths and weaknesses. There are, of course, other interview tips. I have included this list to present some general ideas about your presentations:

- You should dress to impress. Whether you are male or female, you should definitely wear a suit. I have seen people show up at interviews wearing khaki pants and a polo shirt and they look uncomfortable and completely out of place. Do not let that happen to you! Dress as nicely as possible and groom yourself appropriately. Remember you are selling yourself, so you want to look your best.

- Bring a notepad and pen. Ask if you can take notes, and then jot down ideas while still maintaining eye contact. This will show you are interested in what they have to say.

- Do not chew gum! Instead, keep some breath mints in your pocket.

- Look the interviewer in the eye. Try to concentrate on what they are saying and demonstrate that you are interested in what they have to say.

- Shake hands at the beginning of the interview when you introduce yourself. Pay attention to the interviewer's name. After the interview, thank them for their time by using their name (if you need to, jot it down on your notepad!).

- Smile during the interview and appear enthusiastic about the program.

- Do not act inappropriately or immature. Enough said.

- Arrive on time. In fact, commit to arriving 15-20 minutes early! If you are traveling long distances to get there, make arrangements to be early. Use a map program to provide clear directions. The last thing you want to do is show up late, demonstrating that you do not appreciate their time.

- If you are very nervous, it is ok to tell the interviewer that. If you think your anxiety will seriously affect how you interview, it is ok to tell the interviewer, "I'm feeling a little bit nervous and excited today." While the interviewer may or may not take this into account, at least you have covered your bases.

- As the interview ends, ask for contact information or a business card from each person. Then, send a thank you card to those people you met with and interviewed with, letting them know were grateful to have the opportunity to meet with them in person.
- If you do not have additional time constraints, visit the city and the neighborhood either the day before or the day after the interview. You are already there, so make the most of your trip. You might not get another chance, because of time or financial limitations, to revisit all of the locations again.

The bottom line: this may be your only opportunity to go to the school, meet the faculty, and see the facilities before you make a school decision. Make the most of this opportunity! It is your job to promote yourself and to explain why they should choose you and not Jim or Jane Doe who look exactly like you do on paper. Practice answering questions beforehand, smile, and finally **remember to relax.**

Getting In, Waiting, or Trying Again

The PA application process can be lengthy, time-consuming, expensive, and emotionally exhausting. However, like all things in life, the end will arrive at some point. The application process will end in one of three ways: acceptance, wait-listing, or rejection.

Acceptance

If you are accepted to a PA program, fantastic! You are finished with the stresses associated with the application process. If you have been accepted, be sure to make the necessary deposit payment on time in order to reserve your spot in the program. As you did before, send your check with a return receipt requested.

If you have been accepted to one PA program, but are still waiting to hear back from your first choice school, you are in a difficult position. In this case, you may have to pay the deposit to guarantee your spot in at least one program, or risk not having a spot at any PA program. Unfortunately, this happened to me. I had to pay the $500 deposit to hold my spot in the first PA program I was accepted to, while waiting to find out if I had gotten into my first choice. The idea of a school making you pay this fee is frustrating, but they need to know quickly whether or not you are going to matriculate into their program (and, to clarify, not all PA programs will make you pay a deposit to hold your spot). Most PA programs have many students waiting to get in – so if you decide to relinquish your spot, they will give it away to another student. If you do matriculate into a PA program, the deposit you pay goes towards your tuition. However, if you have paid the fee and do not end up attending the PA program, the fee will not be refunded. Make sure you budget for this potential "hidden" cost.

Wait-listing

If you have been wait-listed, do not worry. You have joined a long and distinguished group of students. Wait-listing is what PA schools do when they have offered most of their spots to applicants, but are still waiting to find out if those applicants will matriculate into the program. While being wait-listed is disappointing, it does mean that you are still being considered for a spot.

If you have been wait-listed, I suggest you send a letter to the PA program demonstrating your continued desire to be a part of their program and explain why you believe you are a good fit. You should mention any activities you are currently participating in (e.g. volunteering or taking a biology course) that may further demonstrate your commitment to the profession. Take this opportunity to augment your application with new, pertinent information that may not have been available when you first applied. You may also want to consider having another letter of recommendation sent in. Not all programs will actually use these items to help make their decision as to whether or not you gain admission, but it will not hurt to try, and these actions will only potentially benefit you.

If you have been wait-listed, and have been accepted at another PA program, maybe you should consider releasing your spot on the wait-list. If you think you will be just as happy going to PA school somewhere that has already accepted you, then go there. Additionally, this will free up a spot for someone else who is likely on that school's wait-list. Do not stress yourself out waiting to hear back from the school that wait-listed you. My advice is to pay the deposit and move on with your life. And, be happy you are going to PA school and do not have to worry about the application process anymore!

Rejection

If you have been rejected, it is not the end of the world. You may be wondering, what do I do now? Well, you have a few different options. First of all, you should rethink the decision as to whether or not you really want to be a PA. Do you really want to go through the application process again? As a personal decision, is it worth it to you? If you choose to abandon the PA profession, I wish you well in whatever career endeavors you pursue. However, if you decide you still want to become a PA, you have to go through this entire process again. Take a moment to reflect, and take a deep breath, but then re-motivate yourself. Get excited.

First, I suggest you call the schools that did not accept you and ask them specifically why you did not get in. Be professional, not confrontational. Find out what the reason was. Was your GPA too low? Did they think you needed more healthcare experience? Did you interview poorly? Whatever it is, you need to find out so that you can work on that specifically in anticipation for the next round of applications.

Focus on making yourself a stronger applicant this second time around. You have been through the process once, so you have a terrific idea of what you can expect. Carefully go through this book and see if there was anything you missed. Consider alternative PA programs. Since you will have some extra time, try to get more healthcare experience. Contact the PA you shadowed before and ask if you can shadow him or her again. Take a certification course – possibly a nursing assistant course or an EMT course. Join a PA organization and attend a conference where you can network with PAs and educators from different locations.

Whatever you do, work on improving your application. You need to show the schools you are applying to that you really want to be a PA, and that you will do whatever it takes to become one. You may even want to talk about your initial rejection in your personal statement. If being rejected from PA school influenced you to want to try even harder to get in, then you may want to share that experience with the programs you are applying to. PA programs will want to know what you have done to make yourself a stronger applicant if you were rejected once before.

Just remember that whatever happens, whether you are accepted or rejected, you will still be the same person that you were before. These may sound like empty platitudes, but no matter what the outcome is, you will still have the same drive and the same desire to help people, and if being a PA was not meant for you, there are plenty of other great careers you can pursue.

Physician Assistant School in a Nutshell

Most physician assistant programs are about two to three years in length and are divided into two separate parts: the didactic portion and the clinical portion. The two parts are quite different in terms of what and how you will be learning.

The didactic portion

The didactic portion of any PA school is by far the most challenging part for most students. In fact, this is the part of the program that many students fail to make it through. Most programs are set up so that students have class all day long, from 8 a.m. until 6 or 7 p.m., commonly with three or four exams per week. This means that, after a long day in the classroom or laboratory, you must study for several hours each night in order to try to retain the information. It can be overwhelming. The expectations for you as a PA student are extremely high, and in order to survive the program, you have to find a way to make school your number one priority.

Try to pay attention in class. In PA school, students are typically presented with large volumes of information in lecture format. I know it is easy to "zone out" during lectures, to play on your computer, or to send text messages to your friends. However, it is your responsibility to learn all of the core principles of medicine during this short didactic period before beginning clinical rotations. Paying attention in class can make learning these principles much easier. Try to think of your brain as a sponge, and its purpose is to absorb as much of the information as it possibly can. You will, inevitably, forget information that you have learned along the way, but if you make an effort to pay attention in class and soak up as much as you can, you will have an easier time recalling information when you actually need it.

Some people study well in groups. If you believe you are one of these people, form a study group with some of your classmates. Each of you can take on certain topics and teach them to the other members of the group. Or, each of you can type up summaries of lectures for easier group and individual study. If you do not like to study in groups, find another method that works for you. Maybe you need to go to a quiet place like the library each night for a few hours. Maybe you need to make note-cards for yourself. Find out what works for you and stick to it. Just remember that, above all, consistency is key.

When students struggle with the didactic portion of the PA program curriculum, this can impact nearly everything in their lives. Stress affects people in different ways, and you will need to find a way to balance the stress in your life as a PA student. For me, working out each day was a great way for me to deal with my stress. I would even study while walking on the treadmill or the elliptical. Whatever you do, remember to take care of yourself. Make sure you eat properly and try to get as much sleep as you can. If you are having trouble managing the stress, speak to someone at your program about it. They will likely be able to find you help if you need it.

Sometimes the competition among PA students can be very intense. Most PA students are extremely intelligent, and they may be used to obtaining high marks in school. In nearly every PA program, there will be students who naturally excel when it comes to tests and grades. While it is important to do well in school, try hard to ignore the competition. You are in PA school to learn. So, try to do the best that you can without allowing your grades and the grades of your peers to upset you. Remember, when PA school is over and done, it will be you and your patient alone in the exam room, not you, your patient, and your classmates. Doing your personal best, as long as you pass, is all that will matter in the long run.

The best advice I can give you for surviving the didactic portion is to stay organized. Try to decide what is most important in terms of studying and manage your time wisely. You will never regret being well-prepared. You may also consider asking the faculty to help you stay organized – especially the course director or preclinical coordinator. These people have plenty of experience, and they are dedicated to helping you succeed in the program.

During the didactic portion you will have books that are required for your courses. Find out if any of the upperclassmen are willing to sell or share their books with you before you purchase them all on your own. It is also a good idea to ask your peers or colleagues which books they have found particularly useful before purchasing.

I have created a list of some of my favorite books for use during the didactic portion of PA school:

- **Color Atlas of Anatomy: A Photographic Study of the Human Body**, by Johannes W. Rohen
- **Cecil Essentials of Medicine**, by Thomas E. Andreoli
- **Lippincott's Illustrated Reviews: Pharmacology: Special Millennium Update**, by Mary Julia Mycek
- **Surgical Recall**, By Lorne H. Blackbourne
- **Rapid Interpretation of EKG's**, by Dale Dubin
- **Tarascon Pocket Pharmacopoeia**, by Steven M. Green
- **Physiology (Board Review Series)**, by Linda S. Costanzo
- **Current Medical Diagnosis & Treatment**, by Lawrence M. Tierney
- **Maxwell Quick Medical Reference**, by Robert W. Maxwell

There also several great series of books on medical and surgical topics. Below are some of the most helpful book series for studying and test-taking your didactic year:

- The Blueprints Series
- Appleton and Lange Practice Questions
- Made Ridiculously Simple Series
- The Secrets Series

The clinical portion

Once you get to the clinical portion of the program, you have made it through the first gauntlet. Clinical rotations are in no way easy, but the stress of a clinical rotation is much more physical than it is mental – and most people appreciate that. Most schools have you participate in rotations that are approximately 4-8 weeks long. Each rotation will be a different specialty: for example, you may spend your first rotation doing family practice, and your next rotation doing general surgery. There are some rotations that you are required to do, and others that you may choose to participate in.

What you will actually be doing for each varies from rotation to rotation. Sometimes you will be working the dayshift, and other times you will be working night shifts. Try to adapt the best that you can. Most hospital rotations will include some type of morning rounds, followed by floor-work (drawing blood, ordering tests, etc…) or actually spending time in the operating room. If you are working in an outside clinic, you will likely be examining patients all day. Again, each rotation is unique in that it provides you with a different type of training, in a different setting, with different hours and responsibilities.

Some rotations will require you to travel great distances, which can make your day seem even longer. During my surgery rotation, I had to be at the hospital by 5 a.m. to "pre-round" on my patients. Because my rotation was so far away, I had to leave my house around 3:30 a.m. in order to be on time. Unfortunately, this is not abnormal. You can expect to work long hours on your clinical rotations.

When I was a student doing a surgical rotation, I did not know what to expect. The first day of my first surgical rotation, I was told to scrub into a case in the operating room. Excitedly, I scrubbed in and gowned up just as I had learned in my PA class beforehand. What I was not prepared for, however, was the fact that the operation would last nearly six hours! About three hours into the case, I began to feel a little bit light-headed. I had never fainted before, so I thought I would be fine. A few minutes later, I felt even worse.

The next thing I remember the nurses were putting oxygen on me and putting me into a bed in the recovery room. I had fainted in the operating room. While this is extremely embarrassing, it is not uncommon. PA students and medical students who are not used to being in the operating room for long periods of time are much more likely to get sick. However, you can prepare yourself. The secret is to keep a snack in your labcoat pocket and a beverage in your bag at all times. You never know when you will get a chance to eat on rotations, and having something handy can prevent you from getting sick or getting lightheaded.

If a hospital gives you anything to use while you are there, like a pager or a PDA, I suggest you take very good care of it. You need not guard it with your life, but do treat it like your own. When I was a student, one of the hospitals required me to use their pager in addition to my own. One day, while I was going to the bathroom with my labcoat on the pager fell out of my pocket and into the toilet just as I flushed. My preceptors were very kind once they stopped laughing. Unfortunately, I did have to pay for a replacement pager because I had lost the original. So, be careful with other peoples' property. If you damage it or lose it, you will likely have to pay for it.

Terminology

There are some terms you should be familiar with before you begin your rotations. The first is "pimping." First guesses aside, pimping students on hospital rounds is actually the questioning practice physicians (and PAs) use to force students to be prepared and to think quickly. Attending physicians typically pimp medical and PA students by asking them obscure questions while expecting students to respond with correct answers. I honestly believe that when people pimp students they think they are helping to teach them something; however, I personally feel that this method of making someone feel stupid because they do not remember exact details is not necessarily the best way to teach.

Another term you should be familiar with is "scutwork," because as a PA student, you will definitely do your fair share of scutwork. Scutwork refers to a number of patient care activities that offer very little educational value for the student. For example, a PA student is doing scutwork if he is sent to deliver bloods to the lab, asked to transport a patient to another floor, or told to make phone calls for a resident or intern. Oftentimes they are tasks that need to be done in order to facilitate patient care, but tasks that offer very little in terms of learning experiences. Hopefully, when you are a PA student, you will not be doing much scutwork. However, if you find yourself in a position where you are getting plenty of scutwork but very little substantive experience, bring it to the attention of your program's administrators. Remember – you are paying to learn.

Spending long hours on your feet during rotations will require you to purchase a pair of good shoes. Regardless of your budget, it will not take long before you find yourself willing to eat the expense of quality foot-wear. You may already have a personal preference when it comes to shoes, and if you do that is fine. Most people I know wear tennis shoes or special orthopaedic shoes. If you are looking to purchase a great (but expensive) pair of shoes, my colleagues recommend the following brands: Dansko, Ecco, Birkenstock, and Merrell. I recommend investing in at least one good pair of shoes for your rotations – if for nothing else in this book, you will someday thank me for this advice.

Try to make the best of your rotations; after all, this is the only clinical experience you are going to get before you are working on your own. If someone offers to teach you something, take them up on it. You should never refuse an opportunity to learn something new. As an example, a friend of mine attending physician assistant school made an effort to keep in touch with the medical and surgical residents in some of the hospitals after he had finished his rotation. The residents informed him of any unique cases they had, and because of his curiosity and willingness to learn, he ended up seeing a lot of great medical and surgical cases.

If you have a great attitude, and you are willing to get your hands wet (or dirty), you can learn an incredible amount on your clinical rotations. The best mantra I can give you about your rotations is: be on time, work hard, smile, read if you have downtime, and **do not whine!**

Finally, also write down contact information for physicians and other healthcare professionals whose company or work styles you enjoy. Even though I sound like a skipping CD, you may need letters of recommenda-tion in the future, or you may want to network professionally. Keep your contact list current! PA school is tough, but once you complete your first rotation, you can complete them all – and you can certainly finish the program.

After you have completed your PA education, you will have many decisions to make about which path you would like to take as a professional. You may decide to continue your training, or you may decide to begin working as a PA. Either way, you will have to become certified in order to fully complete your path to practicing as a PA.

Residencies and fellowships

After you become a PA graduate, you will have the option of obtaining additional training in a specialized area of practice by completing a residency or fellowship. Some new graduates believe they can obtain the skills through work experience, while others prefer to gain further experience through organized training programs. Almost all postgraduate training programs are organized to be intense, allowing the participant a great deal of experiences in a condensed period of time. Most postgraduate programs can be completed in 12-15 months, and these programs often provide a salary or stipend.

There are a number of excellent residencies and fellowships available for physician assistants. As of now, there are residencies for PAs in the following specialties: cardiothoracic surgery, critical care, dermatology, emergency medicine, hospitalist, neonatology, neurology, neurosurgery, OB-GYN, oncology, orthopaedics surgery, psychiatry, rheumatology, sleep medicine, surgery, trauma and urology.

There are also teaching fellowships available for PAs that want to gain experience for a career in academia. I detail many of the residencies and fellowships at the end of this book – please consult the indices.

Becoming certified

In order to practice as a PA, you must become a PA-C (physician assistant – certified). In order to do this, you must take and successfully pass the Physician Assistant National Certifying Exam (PANCE). The PANCE is a computerized, multiple-choice test that all PAs must take. The exam is made up of 360 questions that cover topics in both medicine and surgery. The PANCE is very difficult, and it will require you to study a great deal beforehand.

While you are a student in PA school, you will likely take two separate "practice PANCEs" called "ePackrats" or "mock" board exams. These exams are taken at your school, along with your classmates, and they help assess your level of knowledge. You will likely take your ePackrat or mock board exams twice during your time as a student: once before you begin clinical rotations, and once again before you graduate. These exams are similar to the PANCE, in that they are computerized and multiple choice. Getting comfortable taking examinations on the computer will only enhance your ability to do well on the PANCE.

To find out the most up to date information about the PANCE, check out their website: http://www.nccpa.net.

In order to help students study for the PANCE, the NCCPA has designed "blueprints" to guide you. The blueprints can be found on the website, and the blueprints show a breakdown of the content on the exam. For example, approximately 16% of the exam questions will deal with history taking and performing physical examinations. Once you have reviewed the blueprints, you will know what information you need to study.

There are several great study guides out there for the PANCE exam, but I must warn you that some of the programs are very costly. Remember to include these costs in your budget for school as well. You may want to consider sharing books or programs with classmates to save money.

While every student studies differently, I personally found that working through practice questions was the best way for me to learn. If you think this is how you would like to study, consider purchasing the Kaplan Q bank online (http://www.kaplanmedical.com), and/or the Datachem software for PAs (https://www.certistep.com/index.asp). You will also want to use old exams from the ePackrat and books such as Appleton and Lange Review for the Physician Assistant, and A Comprehensive Review for the Certification and Recertification Examinations for Physician Assistants.

Despite the extremely high cost, some students also take review courses before taking the PANCE. The most common review course is put on by CME Resources, and most people I have spoken with were quite happy with it. You can find out more information about that course at: http://www.cmeresources.com.

Continuing Medical Education

In order to maintain your credentialing as a PA after you complete school, you are required to obtain continuing medical education (CME) credits. Currently, the NCCPA requires every PA to obtain 100 CME credit hours every 2 years, broken into 50 hours of category I credits and 50 hours of category II credits. This means that you will have to continue to read journals, attend conferences, or take certification courses to maintain your status as a PA. This is not at all unusual, as most professions require you to obtain some sort of continuing education to continue to work. Once you begin these activities, make a new folder (yes, another folder) and keep all of your certificates together.

You can log your activities either online or on paper, but I recommend a paper copy regardless. The NCCPA does have the right to audit you at any time, so be sure to have paper documentation of any CME credit hours you obtain in case you need to present these to the NCCPA. You can find out more information about CME requirements at the NCCPA website, currently online at:
http://www.nccpa.net/CME_requirements.aspx.

Recertification

Practicing PAs need to take a recertification exam every six years. This exam is called the Physician Assistant National Recertifying Exam (PANRE). Most people study for the PANRE the same way they studied for the PANCE. The PANRE is currently offered in two formats: online and take-home. However, they will phase out the take-home recertification exam by 2010. As you are just applying to PA school, this is likely of little importance to you, so I will avoid any detail. If you would like more information about the PANRE, you can check the NCCPA website.

Working as a physician assistant

So, you are done with school and you have passed the PANCE. Now you need a job! It is an exciting time to be a PA, as the opportunities for you in the workforce are absolutely endless. Nowadays, PAs work in almost every specialty imaginable, such as burn surgery, cardiothoracic surgery, colorectal surgery, critical care, emergency medicine, family practice, general surgery, head and neck, ear nose and throat, neurosurgery, ophthalmology, oncology, orthopaedic surgery, pediatrics, plastic surgery, transplant surgery, urology, interventional radiology, and so on. That is one of the great aspects of being a PA: you do not have to specialize in one specific area.

You should probably begin looking for jobs a few months prior to graduation. However, it is ok if you would prefer to wait until you have passed your board exam to begin your search. I know several people who had jobs before graduation, as well as many others who waited until they became a PA-C. When to begin job-hunting is completely up to you, determined only by your time and budget preferences.

There are several ways to find jobs. You may find a job through a posting online, through a previous rotation, through a PA journal, or even through word of mouth. When I first began to look for jobs, I used the internet to search certain websites daily. Here are just a few of what I believe are the most useful PA job websites currently available:

PA World www.paworld.net. This is the most comprehensive job website I have found. The easiest way to navigate this site is to search for jobs by date. Select the most current date and a website will pop-up with all of the current listings across the country. This website is updated daily, so I recommend book-marking it and checking it frequently.

PA Job Link – Health-e-careers www.aapa.org. This website is sponsored in part by the AAPA, and you can find a link to this page at the AAPA website. This is also a great website for nationwide jobs and it is frequently updated.

AASPA website www.aaspa.com. The AASPA website has job postings specifically for surgical PAs. Check frequently as updates are posted on a weekly basis.

Do not forget to check for job postings at your PA program, as former students often inform their PA programs of job openings. And, if you are looking for a job in a different state than the location of your current PA school, consider contacting PA schools near where you hope to work. They just might be able to put you in touch with the right person.

Also, check your state-sponsored PA organization's website. I have found these websites very useful for finding jobs locally. Oftentimes you must be a member of the organization in order to view the job postings, but if you are going to be living in that area you should consider joining anyway.

You can also check hospital websites to look for jobs. If you know you want to work at a certain hospital, drop off a resume at that hospital and ask them to keep it on file. Finally, do not overlook the importance of going to CME meetings and networking! At every CME conference, there is plenty of time between lectures to meet new PAs and to make possible employment connections.

Physician assistant salaries

Obviously, salary is one of the most important parts of a job (while you may really wish to help, most PA jobs do not expect you to work for free). According to the 2007 AAPA census information, the average new graduate salary for a physician assistant is $71,825. This is the national average, so it varies by both geographic location and by specialty. Know your particular location and situation – before you begin interviewing, you should have an idea of what type of salary you are expecting.

Bargaining for a higher salary can be tough as a new graduate. If you are taking a job at a hospital, it is almost impossible to bargain because hospitals usually have a payscale that only increases based on experience. However, if you are working in a private practice you can bargain for whatever you think you are worth. As I write this, if I were a new graduate I would not accept a full-time job (40 hours or more) that offered a salary of less than $70,000 per year. If someone offers you less than that for a full-time PA position, you should bargain. According to current figures, you are worth at least that much!

If you have an offer in hand, you might show the person or organization extending the offer the national and state averages for salaries during your negotiations. You can get this information online at the Advance PA Magazine website: http://physician-assistant.advanceweb.com. You can also purchase a customized salary report from the AAPA at: http://www.aapa.org/joblink/candidates.html. If your employer cannot budge on salary, consider bargaining for premium-paid health coverage, gym membership, a company car, or other perks in lieu of actual salary dollars. Do not talk yourself out of a job, but be your own best advocate.

Creating a resume

Creating a resume is an important task in getting a job. A resume is the first glimpse that a physician or hospital has to decide whether or not they want to invite you for an interview, and you do not want to be denied an interview simply because your resume was poorly done.

Great resumes are clear and simple. As a new graduate, your resume should be limited to one page. After you have experience as a PA (or if you have an extensive work history before becoming a PA), your resume may exceed one page. Your first PA resume should include the following information:

- Name
- Contact information (make sure it is current)
- Education
- Work experience
- PA school rotations
- Certifications
- Extracurricular activities (optional)

As a new graduate, you should be able to get some help with your resume from your PA program's career services department (or the parent school's). There are also PA organizations that will offer to help you with your resume. For example, the AASPA offers a free resume critique service for new PAs. To contact them about this, visit their website at: www.aaspa.com and search for "resume." The AAPA also offers information about creating resumes and cover letters. The AAPA website resume website is: http://www.aapa.org/joblink/candidates.html.

Interviewing for your first job

Interviewing for your first job as a physician assistant can be stressful. Most schools offer general help with resumes and interviews, but they may not cover specific details. I have reviewed some important ideas below:

You should begin by thinking about your skills and your interests. You should have truthful answers prepared to commonly asked questions:

- Why do you want to work in this setting?
- What can you offer the hospital/practice (skills, research interests, etc...)?
- What are your strengths?
- What are your weaknesses?

Practicing answers to these questions out loud will allow you to be more confident when you are actually interviewing.

The guidelines you followed when you interviewed for PA school should also be followed when interviewing for a PA job. When you begin the actual interview, be sure you are dressed appropriately. You should wear a suit and appear well groomed. Greet the interviewer with a firm hand-shake and try to maintain eye contact throughout the interaction. It is also a good idea to observe the setting as you walk through the hospital or office. Is it clean and welcoming? Do you feel comfortable in the environment? Does the staff appear pleasant? Could you see yourself working there?

You may run into a question that you are not sure how to answer. If that happens, just as you did during PA school interviews, be polite and simply tell the interviewer that you are not sure. Be honest! The interviewer knows you are a new graduate; therefore, he will not expect you to know everything.

You should also be prepared to ask about the job and the setting. Consider asking the following questions:

- What will my role be in this setting?
- What will my responsibilities be outside of patient care?
- What is a typical work day like?
- Will I work in one hospital/clinic or will I be working at satellite offices?
- Will the job require me to be on call?
- Will there be an opportunity for professional growth?

Most interviewers will not bring up salary on the first interview. Be prepared to ask about the salary range, malpractice insurance, and benefits when you return for a follow-up interview.

At the end of the interview, make sure you establish clear communication regarding a potential follow-up. Will you contact them if you are interested, or will they contact you? If they will contact you, how long should it take? Finally, ask if there is more information that you can provide to help assist their consideration.

Once you have landed a job

Starting your first job as a PA, regardless of your past work experiences, can be both exciting and scary. During your first year of work experience, you will almost certainly learn a significant amount. You will grow as a clinician by making mistakes and by learning from those mistakes. I have listed some "first-job" advice below.

- **As a practicing PA, you are responsible for everything you do.** If you make a mistake, it is your responsibility to own up to it. If you forgot to order a test or if you overlooked an abnormal lab result, admit you made the mistake and move on. In a perfect world, we would not make mistakes – but we are human and unfortunately, we do make mistakes. The sooner you admit you have done something wrong, the sooner you (and possibly others) can try to fix the mistake. Do not postpone notifying others if you do make a mistake – timing may be an important component of fixing even a life-threatening error. Just remember to learn from your mistakes after they have been corrected.

- **Always have someone available to contact who can help you when you need help.** There will be times when you have no idea what is wrong with your patient, or how exactly to treat your patient. When this happens, you need to call for help. Whether you call your attending physician, a senior PA, or even a resident – sometimes it is best to call someone else and notify them of what exactly is happening and why you are concerned. My personal belief is that it never hurts to inform those who are working above you. They should know what is going on, and if they are good practitioners they will want to know and will want to assist you.

- **Listen to the nurses.** You should always listen to what the nurses are saying. They spend much more time with the patients than you do, so if they are concerned about something – you must pay attention to them. However, you do not always have to do what the nurses ask you to do (i.e. order a medication or test that you do not believe is appropriate). Take their recommendations into consideration, but remain the responsible party.

- **Document everything neatly.** If you took the time to see the patient, take the time to write your note legibly so that others can read it. I cannot tell you how many times I have looked in a chart and been unable to identify anything that a doctor, PA, or NP has written. Communicating with other services is a huge part of our jobs. Be responsible and make sure you write your orders and notes legibly so that others know what exactly you were thinking when you saw your patient. Also, remember it is a legal document and could be scrutinized during an inquiry or litigation.

Promoting yourself as a physician assistant

I have explained what a PA is to many more people than I can remember. Our profession is over 40 years old, yet many people I have met still have no idea what a PA is. That means it is important for all of us to promote ourselves as physician assistants and to make good impressions for the profession. If you work in a small hospital and are the only PA, you need to work hard to make a name for future physician assistants in your hospital. If you have made a bad impression in your hospital, it is possible that they will not hire another PA after you are gone.

While physician assistants receive little training in topics related to business, it is necessary to know how to "market" yourself. Marketing yourself simply means identifying what you are good at and emphasizing those skills. When it comes to clinical skills, it is important to document some of your skills. For example, if you have first assisted in 50 laparoscopic cholecystectomies, then you know how to do this case in the operating room.

If you know what you have done, when interview for your next job, you can explain exactly what you have done and sell yourself in that fashion. Many physicians who have never had a PA before do not realize how valuable you really are. If you can sell yourself well, you can land any job. Part of recognizing your skills is listing what you have done. Keep a brief journal or list of your tasks, and you will always remember your experiences. Keep your resume updated as well.

Another important aspect of promoting yourself as a PA is being able to network with other healthcare professionals. These networking skills will help you throughout your career to find new opportunities for both work and further learning. Always take the time to meet people and to get their contact information by requesting a business card, following up with an e-mail address, or by taking down everything longhand. You never know when a contact may come in handy.

Paying off your debt

As someone who gradated from PA school with an incredible amount of student loan debt, I can tell you that paying back student loans is not fun. In fact, many students have over six figures of student loan debt. While PA salaries are good, they are still not high enough to pay back the loans as quickly as you might want to.

For my student loans, I ended up putting about half of my monthly salary towards the loans. If I had any extra money or received a refund from my taxes, I always put the money towards my student loans. And, when paying back the loans, it makes basic financial sense to first pay down the higher interest private loans. The sooner you can get rid of the private loans, with their higher attendant interest rates, the better.

Also, please do not compromise your retirement account (401k, 403b, or IRA) to pay off your loans. It is just as important to put money away for retirement as it is to pay off your loans. Instead, you may have to cut back on the fun type of purchases, like fancy cars and vacations. Remember how you got used to living frugally as a student? Unfortunately, that does not end immediately after school. When you are a practicing PA, you will probably have to be careful with money for a few more years – at least until you get ahead on your student loans.

Before you begin working, or even interviewing, you should have an understanding of some of the current laws regarding professional practice and how they will apply to you and how you will provide patient care. Some of these issues will arise during your interviews, and, if you are at a loss for interesting essay topics, you may be able to combine one of the topics below with your personal experience to show how your interests intersect with important current PA issues.

Prescription rights for physician assistants

As of 2007, all fifty states, including the District of Columbia and Guam, have prescribing rights. Each state or territory has its own specific laws as to what PAs are able to prescribe. You will need to check out the specific requirements for both where you matriculate and where you practice. Much of this information is available online. Please visit the AAPA website at: http://www.aapa.org for details.

Physician assistant working relationships

The working relationship between a physician and a physician assistant varies depending on the setting and the personalities of the people involved, but the relationship should always be based on mutual trust and respect. Ultimately, while the physician is responsible for the care of the patient, the PA still plays a large role in the way that care is provided.

When I was a PA student, I quickly learned that I should always "know my limits" when practicing professionally. As a PA, you may be able to function like a physician in many situations, but you always need to know when to ask for help. If you do not feel comfortable performing a procedure or are unsure of the appropriate treatment for a patient, always ask your supervising physician for help. These questions are within your scope of practice, and should be encouraged. A close working relationship between the physician and the physician assistant ultimately allows for better delivery of patient care.

Some PAs experience a great deal of autonomy within their work-setting. The amount of autonomy you have in your job will depend both upon the setting and your relationship with your physician. Again, no matter what the level of autonomy, the physician must always be available for consultation with the PA. This consultation can occur in person or via some method of telecommunication (phone, e-mail, pagers, etc…). Some PAs work in clinics where their supervising physician is never in person, so these PAs act as the sole provider. However, because PAs are always subject to physician supervision, this type of work environment is only possible when the supervising physician has made arrangements to be available for contact at any time of day. PAs who work in this type of setting experience a great deal of autonomy and responsibility, but they must not forget the extent of their scope of practice.

Other PAs work directly with their supervising physician throughout the day. These PAs actually see patients together with their physician and participate in procedures together. As long as you are working within the scope of practice designated by your supervising physician, you are doing your job appropriately.

How comfortable you are with direct responsibility should impact your job search. If you desire autonomy and enjoy responsibility, consider practices with remote supervision. If you are more comfortable taking direction and cues from a physician, make sure you work in a supervised environment. And, always remember the cardinal rule for PA practice: **the physician must be available for consult.**

Physician assistant reimbursement

In order for PAs to be useful in the clinical setting, we must be cost-effective. As physician assistants we can provide high quality patient care somewhat independent of physicians, and we can reduce the cost of delivering that care. Over the years, various PA organizations have worked very hard to help create laws that allow us to be reimbursed by private insurance companies, Medicare, and Medicaid for the services we provide. This discussion may seem premature, but this topic may come up during PA school interviews, and it is a great subject to demonstrate the depth of your interest in becoming a PA.

Reimbursement from private insurance companies usually provides for the services provided by PAs as long as those services are included as part of the physician's bill. The amount they cover will vary from insurance company to insurance company, and from state to state.

Physician assistants also receive reimbursement from Medicaid programs for services provided. As of now, all 50 states will provide reimbursement for amounts that are either the same amount as or slightly lower than the customary amounts paid to physicians.

Reimbursement for Medicare services is more complicated. In 1998, the Centers for Medicare and Medicaid Services (CMS) revised its Medicare Carriers Manual reimbursement guidelines to include those services rendered by PAs. Medicare will reimburse for medical services provided by PAs in all settings at 85 percent of the physician's customary fee. However, each state has its own specific laws – therefore, the reimbursement may be affected if services are not provided according to state law.

In 2002, CMS issued new "Medicare Carriers Manual" instructions allowing PAs and physicians to bill at 100 percent of the physician's fee. This law requires that the physician and the PA work for the same employer or practice and share visits made to patients the same day. This means that the physician must actually spend some "face-time" with the patient in order for the PA's service to be billed at 100 percent of the physician's fee. If the physician does not provide "face-time," the PAs patient visit may only be billed at the PA's fee of 85 percent. It is more lucrative for a physician to be on-site and seeing patients with the PA; however, for some physicians, billing at the PA's fee of 85 percent is just as profitable because it gives the physician time to participate in other aspects of patient care.

There is another way services provided by a PA can be billed at 100 percent of the physician's fee. This provision of the law is called "incident-to" and applies to outpatient services that are provided in offices and clinics. There are three specific guidelines that must be followed in order for the services to be billed at the physician's fee:

- The physician must be on site when the PA is providing care
- The physician must treat all new (first-visit) Medicare patients
- The physician must treat all established Medicare patients with a new medical condition.

Medicare has very specific guidelines for reimbursement, and it is important for billing purposes that the guidelines are properly followed.

Physician Assistants who work in the operating room as first assistants have slightly different reimbursement guidelines. Medicare provides reimbursement for a physician who first assists in the operating room at a rate of 16 percent of the primary surgeon's fee. When a PA first assists in the operating room, the billing percentage is less. The PA first assistant is reimbursed for 85 percent of the physician's first assistant rate of 16 percent, which means the PA first assistant will be reimbursed 13.6 percent of the primary surgeon's fee.

As a PA, providing patient care is typically your most important duty. However, you must pay attention to billing as well. Reimbursement may be affected by improper billing, so PAs must learn to properly bill for their services. In order to bring revenue into a practice or hospital, a physician assistant must accurately bill for the services provided. Most PA programs will teach you basic concepts regarding how to bill, although, depending on the practice setting, the way you will bill for services will vary. Some private practice settings and hospitals have medical professionals (billing specialists and medical coders) who actually do the billing and coding for the physician and the physician assistant which makes this part of a PA's job much easier.

Reimbursement can be extremely confusing. Even professional PAs sometimes find themselves confused about billing issues. For the most up-to-date information about physician assistant reimbursement, please visit the AAPA website at: www.aapa.org.

Malpractice coverage for physician assistants

As a PA, you will need to make sure you are covered under some type of malpractice insurance. As medical malpractice lawsuits are common, practicing without malpractice insurance will put you at great risk. Physician assistants are increasingly being named in medical malpractice lawsuits, and it is important to take the responsibility for making sure you are protected. Even if you are a dependent practitioner working under a supervising physician, you may still be held accountable for any negligent actions you make.

If you work for a hospital or private practice, it is likely that your employer will pay for your malpractice insurance. Take the time before you start work to review your policy carefully to make sure that it covers you appropriately. In addition to the policy provided by your employer (which typically lists you as a provider under a physician's name), you may want to consider paying for your own personal policy for extra protection. You can oftentimes purchase these policies at reasonable rates.

There are different companies that provide malpractice insurance for physician assistants. However, as of the date of this book's publication, there is only one source of PA malpractice insurance endorsed by the AAPA. It is provided by a company called CM & F. To learn more about this insurance policy, please visit their website at: http://www.pavalue.com.

Future of the Profession

As I have said before, it is a great time to be a PA. Every year our numbers grow and our legal rights to practice improve. Although there are bound to be roadblocks ahead, most of the future looks bright. I firmly believe that our profession will continue to progress, and that opportunities for future PAs will expand as well. With that in mind, here are my impressions of and predictions for that progression for the PA profession:

- **The profession will continue to grow.** As the number of accredited PA programs expands, so will the number of working PAs. The need for mid-level practitioners must continue to grow, as there continues to be a projected shortage of primary care physicians, and the hours a resident physician can work is limited to 80 per week. Physician assistants will continue to fill this gap in both the hospital setting and the private practice setting.
- **Competition for jobs with nurse practitioners will increase.** While the demand for mid-level providers continues to increase and there will be an increase in available jobs, an elevated profile for PAs will bring them into direct competition with NPs. More and more hospitals are lumping the two jobs together when they search for potential employees. Hospitals will employ a "PA or NP" standard form search for certain employment positions, thus intensifying competition for jobs between the two categories. This means that the standards for education and practice in both professions will likely increase to differentiate and promote the skills of both degrees.
- **The need for advanced degrees.** Most PA programs are now providing Master's degrees, and those that do not currently are likely in the process of converting to this standard. There are now also programs that provide Doctoral degrees for physician assistants as well. While I do not see the profession as a whole requiring PAs to obtain advanced degrees, some PAs with an eye towards non-clinical employment opportunities within the profession may choose to pursue this path of higher education. Most NP programs now provide their graduates with Master's degrees and

some even provide their graduates with clinical Doctoral degrees. Physical therapist programs now offer Doctoral degrees to their students as well. While it is not necessary to obtain a Doctoral degree to work as a clinical practitioner, those wishing to pursue employment paths in academia will likely pursue these degrees.

- **The need for specialty training.** As more and more PAs begin to work in medical or surgical specialties, the need for further specialty certification or training opportunities will increase. Hospitals and physicians may begin to require PAs to prove their competency in a certain specialty by providing documentation for course or procedure completion. While there are currently no specialty certification requirements for PAs, I envision that future PAs will need these additional educational or clinical certifications for specialty practice.

- **The need for universal reimbursement.** The future of reimbursement for mid-level providers is uncertain. While PAs have worked hard for the current policies they have regarding reimbursement, private insurance companies still have the right to deny payment for services provided by PAs and NPs based on those companies' sometimes arbitrary standards. PAs must continue to work towards universal reimbursement which would require all private insurance companies to pay for their services.

- **Opportunities to work as a PA abroad.** While U.S.-trained PAs are currently working in England, Scotland and Canada, other countries are also considering adopting the use of PAs. As other parts of the world realize a need for more well-trained healthcare providers, the use of PAs abroad should only continue to grow.

- **The need for competent practitioners will grow.** As of 2009, Medicare will stop paying hospitals to treat "preventable" complications. This means that hospitals will not be reimbursed if a patient develops a complication during their hospital stay that Medicare deems preventable. In response, hospitals are already focusing their efforts on decreasing infections, pressure ulcers, and hospital-acquired injuries. PAs will play an incredibly important role in achieving this goal as primary healthcare providers in the hospital setting, and will gain increased responsibility as cost-effective first lines of defense against these types of complications.

Resources

I highly recommend you check out some of these physician assistant resources, as they contain in depth, useful information on further PA topics:

PA Organizations

American Academy of Physician Assistants. (AAPA)
Website: http//www.aapa.org
Content: The organization created by PAs for PAs. This website has most of what you need to know about becoming a PA and being a PA.

American Academy of Nephrology Physician Assistants
Website: http://www.aanpa.org
Content: Supports the professional growth, development, training, education and networking of PAs within the specialty practice of nephrology.

American Academy of Physician Assistants in Occupational Medicine
Website: http://www.aapa.org/spec/AAPAOM
Content: An educational organization representing PAs who share a common interest and role in the care of the working person, and the prevention of workplace illness and injury.

American Academy Physician Assistants in Allergy Asthma and Immunology
Website: http://www.aapa.org/aai
Content: Committed to the education, growth, and development of PAs in allergy, asthma, & immunology.

American Association of Surgical Physician Assistants. (AASPA)
Website: http://www.aaspa.com
Content: The premiere multi-specialty organization for PAs, PA students, and pre-PA students interested in surgery.

American Society of Endocrine Physician Assistants
Website: http://www.endocrine-pa.com
Content: Dedicated to the education, advancement and placement of
PAs in endocrinology.

Association of Neurosurgical Physician Assistants (ANSPA)
Website: http://www.anspa.org
Content: An organization dedicated to the promotion and development
of Physician Assistants working in Neurological Surgery.

Association of Physician Assistants in Cardiovascular Surgery
(APACVS)
Website: http://www.apacvs.org
Content: The premiere organization representing the interests of
Cardiovascular and Thoracic Surgical Physician Assistants.

Association of Physician Assistants in Cardiology
Website: http://cardiologypa.org
Content: A resource for cardiology PAs and PA students.

Association of Physician Assistants in Obstetrics & Gynecology
Website: http://www.paobgyn.org
Content: The only professional association devoted exclusively to PAs
practicing in women's health.

Association of Physician Assistants in Oncology
Website: http://www.apao.cc
Content: Promotes the utilization of Physician Assistants in the delivery of the best possible care available to people with cancer and related
diseases.

Association of Physician Assistants in Anesthesia
Website: http://www.paanesthesiaworld.us
Content: Resource for PAs working in anesthesia.

Association of Plastic Surgery Physician Assistants (APSPA)
Website: http://www.apspa.net
Content: Dedicated to PAs and students interested in working in plastic
surgery.

Association of Psychiatric Physician Assistants
Website: http://www.psychpa.com
Content: Dedicated to Physician Assistants who work in the area of mental health care.

Naval Association of Physician Assistants
Website: http://www.aapa.org/napa
Content: Devoted to educating the public about the PA profession, seeking legislative and governmental policy changes regarding PAs, and informing those in the profession about national Navy issues.

Physician Assistant Education Association (PAEA)
Website: http://www.paeaonline.org/index.html
Content: The only organization that represents physician assistant educational programs.

Physician Assistants in Orthopaedic Surgery (PAOS)
Website: http://www.paos.org
Content: The national organization that represents physician assistants in orthopaedics and in all orthopaedic employment settings. Its membership also includes physician assistant students and supporters of the profession.

Society of Emergency Medicine Physician Assistants (SEMPA)
Website: http://www.sempa.org/
Content: Represents emergency medicine PAs in the United States and around the world.

Society of Army Physician Assistants
Website: http://www.sapa.org
Content: A civilian organization representing and supporting U.S. Army Physician Assistants, including former, active, retired, reserve and National Guard PAs.

Society of Dermatology Physician Assistants
Website: http://www.dermpa.org
Content: Dedicated to promoting the interests of PAs and students in dermatology.

Society of Physician Assistants in Otorhinolaryngology / Head & Neck Surgery
Website: http://www.entpa.org
Content: Promotes the growth and development of Physician Assistants in the ENT field.

Society of Air Force Physician Assistants
Website: http://www.safpa.org
Content: Dedicated to PAs who work in the Air Force community.

Society for Physician Assistants in Pediatrics
Website: http://www.aapa.org/spec/SPAP
Content: Consists of PAs, PA residents and PA students, as well as affiliate and associate individuals who share a common interest in the art of pediatric medicine.

Society of Physician Assistants Caring for the Elderly
Website: http://www.geri-pa.org
Content: Dedicated to sharing information about practicing geriatric medicine as it relates to Physician Assistants and other health care providers.

Society of Physician Assistants in Rheumatology
Website: http://www.aapa.org/spar
Content: Dedicated to enhancing the health and well being of persons with Rheumatological disorders through the representation and advancement of PA/physician teams.

United Kingdom Association of Physician Assistants (UKAPA)
Website: http://www.ukapa.co.uk
Content: UK Association of physician assistants supports the PA profession in the United Kingdom.

Veteran Affairs Physician Assistant Association
Website: http://www.vapaa.org
Content: Dedicated to promoting the interests of physician assistants employed by the U.S. Department of Veterans Affairs.

Physician Assistant Websites For Fun

Advance Magazine for Physician Assistants
Website: http://physician-assistant.advanceweb.com
Content: Provides PAs with clinical articles, professional news and analysis, practice articles and opinions specifically tailored to PAs needs.

Association of American Medical Colleges
Website: http://www.aamc.org/students/start.htm
Content: A resource for medical students or others considering healthcare careers.

NEWS-Line for Physician Assistants
Website: http://www.news-line.com/?-token.target=home&-token.profession=pa
Content: Provides professional news, informative articles and career openings.

Physician Associate Forum
Website: http://www.physicianassociate.com
Content: A forum designed for Pre-PA students, PA students, and PAs in practice.

Student Academy of the American Academy of Physician Assistants
Website: http://saaapa.aapa.org/index.htm
Content: Provides current information related to being a PA student and the PA profession.

Student-Doctor Forum
Website: http://www.studentdoctor.net/
Content: A forum designed for students interested in healthcare professions.

Student Financial Resources

College Answer: The Planning for College Destination
Website: http://www.collegeanswer.com
Content: Offers pointers on the college admission process from preparation to getting loans. Also provides tools that enable users to analyze the affordability of schools.

Fastweb: Scholarships, Financial Aid, and Colleges
Website: http://www.fastweb.com
Content: The nation's largest, most accurate, and most frequently updated scholarship database online.

FinAid: The SmartStudent Guide to Financial Aid
Website: http://www.finaid.org
Content: Provides information about financing a college education.

Free Application for Federal Student Aid
Website: http://www.fafsa.ed.gov
Content: Provides the application and necessary information to receive federal financial aid.

Great Books to Read

A Kernel in the Pod: The Adventures of a Midlevel Clinician in a Top-level World. By J. Michael Jones.

Getting Into the Physician Assistant School of Your Choice. By Andrew J. Rodican.

Med School Confidential: A Complete Guide to the Medical School Experience: By Students, for Students. By Robert H. Miller and Daniel M. Bissell.

Opportunities in Physician Assistant Careers. By Terence J. Sacks.

Physician Assistant: A Guide to Clinical Practice. 4th Edition. By Ruth Ballweg, Darwin Brown, Edward Sullivan, and Dan Vetrosky.

Physician Assistants in American Medicine. By Roderick S. Hooker and James F. Cawley.

Surgical Recall. By Lorne H. Blackbourne.

The Intern Blues: The Timeless Classic About the Making of a Doctor. By Robert Marion.

I have researched and gathered information on each of the 139 physician assistant programs currently accredited in the United States. Please use this information as only your first step; because PA programs can make changes at any time, you should contact each program you are interested to determine their current admission and tuition fee policies.

Programs in Alabama

University of Alabama at Birmingham
Special focus: Surgical Program
Location: Birmingham, AL
Degree granted: Master's Degree
Phone: 205-934-4605
E-mail: kpeoples@uab.edu
Website: http://main.uab.edu/shrp/default.aspx?pid=77392
Supplemental application: Yes, $25 fee
Number of students accepted into program each year: 30-35
Average GPA: 3.4
GRE: Yes
Length of program: 27 months
Uses CASPA: Yes
Tuition Cost: $48,128 (in-state), $89,796 (out-of-state)

University of South Alabama
Special focus: General
Location: Mobile, AL
Degree granted: Master's Degree
Phone: 251-434-3641
E-mail: pastudies@usamail.usouthal.edu
Website: http://www.southalabama.edu/alliedhealth/pa/index.html
Supplemental application: Yes, $110 fee
Number of students accepted into program each year: 36
Average GPA: 3.5
GRE: Yes
Length of program: 27 months
Uses CASPA: Yes
Tuition Cost: $25,531 (in-state), $68,123 (out-of-state)

Programs in Arkansas

Harding University
Special focus: General
Location: Searcy, AR
Degree granted: Master's Degree
Phone: 501-279-5642
E-mail: paprogram@harding.edu
Website: http://www.harding.edu/paprogram/index.html
Supplemental application: No
Number of students accepted into program each year: 32
Average GPA: 3.5
GRE: Yes
Length of program: 28 months
Uses CASPA: Yes
Tuition Cost: $50,050

Programs in Arizona

Arizona School of Health Sciences
Special focus: General, with special track for Native American students
Location: Mesa, AZ
Degree granted: Master's Degree
Phone: 480-219-6000
E-mail: paprogram@atsu.edu
Website: http://www.atsu.edu/ashs/programs/physician_assistant/index.htm
Supplemental application: No
Number of students accepted into program each year: 67
Average GPA: 3.43
GRE: No
Length of program: 26 months
Uses CASPA: Yes
Tuition Cost: $47,350

Midwestern University
Special focus: General, with specializations in research, clinical, bioethics, or health education
Location: Glendale, AZ
Degree granted: Master's Degree
Phone: 623-572-3215
E-mail: N/A
Website: http://www.midwestern.edu/az%2Dpa/
Supplemental application: No
Number of students accepted into program each year: 86
Average GPA: >2.75
GRE: Yes
Length of program: 27 months
Uses CASPA: Yes
Tuition Cost: $72,313

Programs in California

Charles R. Drew University of Medicine and Science
Special focus: Primary Care
Location: Los Angeles, CA
Degree granted: Bachelor's Degree, or Certificate
Phone: 323-563-5879
E-mail: aaronharris@cdrewu.edu
Website: http://www.cdrewu.edu/cosh/physician_assistant/
physician_assistant.htm
Supplemental application: Yes, $35 fee
Number of students accepted into program each year: 60
Average GPA: N/A
GRE: No
Length of program: 24 months
Uses CASPA: No
Tuition Cost: $25,750

Keck School of Medicine of the University of Southern California
Special focus: Primary Care
Location: Alhambra, CA
Degree granted: Master's Degree
Phone: 626-457-4240
E-mail: uscpa@usc.edu
Website: http://www.usc.edu/schools/medicine/departments/physician_assistant/
Supplemental application: Yes, $35 fee
Number of students accepted into program each year: N/A
Average GPA: 3.0
GRE: Yes
Length of program: 33 months
Uses CASPA: Yes
Tuition Cost: $108,000

Loma Linda University
Special focus: General
Location: Loma Linda, CA
Degree granted: Master's Degree
Phone: 909-558-7295
E-mail: bstocker@sahp.llu.edu
Website: http://www.llu.edu/llu/sahp/pa/
Supplemental application: No
Number of students accepted into program each year: 26
Average GPA: 3.5
GRE: No
Length of program: 24 months
Uses CASPA: Yes
Tuition Cost: $63,750

Riverside County/Riverside Community College
Special focus: Primary Care
Location: Moreno Valley, CA
Degree granted: Certificate, or Associate's Degree
Phone: 951-571-6166
E-mail: pa@rcc.edu
Website: http://www.rcc.edu/academicPrograms/physicianAssistant/
Supplemental application: Yes
Number of students accepted into program each year: 28
Average GPA: N/A
GRE: No
Length of program: 24 months
Uses CASPA: No
Tuition Cost: $16,900

Samuel Merritt College
Special focus: General
Location: Oakland, CA
Degree granted: Master's Degree
Phone: 510-869-6623
E-mail: pharrison@samuelmerritt.edu
Website: http://www.samuelmerritt.edu/physician_assistant
Supplemental application: No
Number of students accepted into program each year: 29
Average GPA: 3.45
GRE: No
Length of program: 27 months
Uses CASPA: Yes
Tuition: $64,146

San Joaquin Valley College
Special focus: Primary Care
Location: Visalia, CA
Degree granted: Associate's Degree
Phone: 559-651-2500 ext. 351
E-mail: monicau@sjvc.edu
Website: http://www.sjvc.edu/programs/programs.php?programID=26
Supplemental application: Yes
Number of students accepted into program each year: 24
Average GPA: 2.8
GRE: No
Length of program: 24 months
Uses CASPA: No
Tuition Cost: $48,930

Stanford University School of Medicine
Special focus: Primary Care
Location: Palo Alto, CA
Degree granted: Certificate, Master's Degree option available
Phone: 650-725-6959
E-mail: pcap-information@lists.stanford.edu
Website: http://pcap.stanford.edu/
Supplemental application: Yes
Number of students accepted into program each year: 50
Average GPA: 3.0
GRE: No
Length of program: 16 months
Uses CASPA: No
Tuition Cost: $23,820 (in-state), $32,820 (out-of-state)

Touro University - California College of Health Sciences
Special focus: Public Health
Location: Vallejo, CA
Degree granted: Master's Degree
Phone: 707-638-5978
E-mail: sdavis@touro.edu
Website: http://www.tu.edu/departments.php?id=42&page=549
Supplemental application: No, only sent to qualified applicants
Number of students accepted into program each year: 40
Average GPA: 3.2
GRE: No
Length of program: 32 months
Uses CASPA: Yes
Tuition Cost: N/A

University of California - Davis
Special focus: Primary Care
Location: Sacramento, CA
Degree granted: Certificate
Phone: 916-734-3551
E-mail: fnppa@ucdavis.edu
Website: http://www.ucdmc.ucdavis.edu/fnppa/
Supplemental application: Yes, $40 fee
Number of students accepted into program each year: 60
Average GPA: >2.7
GRE: No
Length of program: 24 months
Uses CASPA: No
Tuition Cost: $24,736 (in-state), $58,014 (out-of-state)

Western University of Health Sciences
Special focus: Primary Care
Location: Pomona, CA
Degree granted: Master's Degree
Phone: 909-469-5378
E-mail: admissions@westernu.edu
Website: http://www.westernu.edu/xp/edu/cahp/mspas_about.xml
Supplemental application: No, only sent to qualified applicants
Number of students accepted into program each year: 98
Average GPA: 3.2
GRE: No
Length of program: 24 months
Uses CASPA: Yes
Tuition Cost: $53,460

Colorado PA Programs

Red Rocks Community College
Special focus: General
Location: Denver, CO
Degree granted: Certificate, Bachelor's and Master's option available
Phone: 303-914-6386
E-mail: arlene.duran@rrcc.edu
Website: http://www.rrcc.edu/pa/
Supplemental application: Yes
Number of students accepted into program each year: 28
Average GPA: 3.2
GRE: No
Length of program: 24 months
Uses CASPA: No
Tuition Cost: $36,600 (in-state), $44,400 (out-of-state)

University of Colorado at Denver and Health Sciences Center
Special focus: Primary Care Pediatric Medicine
Location: Aurora, CO
Degree granted: Master's Degree
Phone: 303-315-7963
E-mail: chapa-info@uchsc.edu
Website: http://www.uchsc.edu/chapa/
Supplemental application: Yes, $25 fee
Number of students accepted into program each year: 40
Average GPA: 3.6
GRE: Yes
Length of program: 36 months
Uses CASPA: Yes
Tuition Cost: $34,390 (in-state), $71,870 (out-of-state)

Connecticut PA Programs

Quinnipiac University
Special focus: General
Location: Hamden, CT
Degree granted: Master's Degree
Phone: 203-582-8672
E-mail: scott.farber@quinnipiac.edu
Website: http://www.quinnipiac.edu/x781.xml
Supplemental application: No
Number of students accepted into program each year: 40
Average GPA: 3.4
GRE: No
Length of program: 27 months
Uses CASPA: Yes
Tuition Cost: $64,000

Yale University School of Medicine
Special focus: General
Location: New Haven, CT
Degree granted: Master's Degree
Phone: 203-785-2860
E-mail: pa.program@yale.edu
Website: http://info.med.yale.edu/phyassoc/
Supplemental application: No
Number of students accepted into program each year: 32 students
Average GPA: 3.3
GRE: Yes
Length of program: 27 months
Uses CASPA: Yes
Tuition Cost: $52,960

Washington DC PA Programs

George Washington University
Special focus: Community Service
Location: Washington, DC
Degree granted: Master's Degree, Master of Public Health option available
Phone: 202-994-7644
E-mail: paadm@gwumc.edu
Website: http://www.gwumc.edu/healthsci/programs/pa/
Supplemental application: Yes
Number of students accepted into program each year: 51
Average GPA: N/A
GRE: Yes
Length of program: 24 months, or 36 months for MPH option
Uses CASPA: Yes
Tuition Cost: $60,840

Howard University
Special focus: General
Location: Washington, DC
Degree granted: Bachelor's Degree, or Certificate
Phone: 202-806-7536
E-mail: mbarnard@howard.edu
Website: http://www.cpnahs.howard.edu/AHS/Pa/Introduction.htm
Supplemental application: Yes
Number of students accepted into program each year: N/A
Average GPA: >2.5
GRE: No
Length of program: Approximately 4 years
Uses CASPA: No
Tuition Cost: N/A

Delaware PA Programs

Arcadia University
Special focus: General
Location: Newark, DE
Degree granted: Master's Degree
Phone: 302-356-9440
E-mail: daysc@arcadia.edu
Website: http://www.arcadia.edu/academic/default.aspx?id=425
Supplemental application: No
Number of students accepted into program each year: 49
Average GPA: >3.2
GRE: Yes
Length of program: 24 months
Uses CASPA: Yes
Tuition Cost: $77,280

Florida PA Programs

Barry University School of Graduate Medical Sciences
Special focus: Primary Care
Location: Miami Shores, FL, and St. Petersburg, FL
Degree granted: Master's Degree
Phone: 305-899-3249
E-mail: mweiner@mail.barry.edu
Website: http://www.barry.edu/pa/Default.asp
Supplemental application: No
Number of students accepted into program each year: 40, and 24
Average GPA: >3.0
GRE: Yes
Length of program: 27 months
Uses CASPA: Yes
Tuition Cost: $84,000

Miami Dade College
Special focus: Primary Care
Location: Miami, FL
Degree granted: Associate's Degree
Phone: 305-237-4124
E-mail: jhernan7@mdc.edu
Website: http://www.mdc.edu/medical/academic_programs/physician_assistant/
physician.htm
Supplemental application: Yes, $25 fee
Number of students accepted into program each year: N/A
Average GPA: >2.5
GRE: No
Length of program: 24 months
Uses CASPA: No
Tuition Cost: $19,540 (in-state), $28,490 (out-of-state)

Nova Southeastern University
Special focus: General
Location: Fort Lauderdale, FL
Degree granted: Master's Degree
Phone: 954-262-1250 or 1-800-541-6682 x1101
E-mail: marquard@nsu.nova.edu
Website: http://www.nova.edu/pa/
Supplemental application: Yes, $50 fee
Number of students accepted into program each year: 85-90
Average GPA: 3.2
GRE: Yes
Length of program: 27 months
Uses CASPA: Yes
Tuition Cost: $43,500

Nova Southeastern University-Naples
Special focus: General
Location: Naples, FL
Degree granted: Master's Degree
Phone: 239-591-4528 ext. 20
E-mail: jkeena@nsu.nova.edu
Website: http://www.nova.edu/panaples/
Supplemental application: Yes, $50 fee
Number of students accepted into program each year: 60
Average GPA: >2.7
GRE: Yes
Length of program: 27 months
Uses CASPA: Yes
Tuition Cost: $44,000

Nova Southeastern University-Orlando
Special focus: General
Location: Orlando, FL
Degree granted: Master's Degree
Phone: 407-264-5153
E-mail: asantiag@nova.edu
Website: http://www.nova.edu/pa/orlando/
Supplemental application: Yes, $50 fee
Number of students accepted into program each year: 50
Average GPA: >2.7
GRE: Yes
Length of program: 27 months
Uses CASPA: Yes
Tuition Cost: $43,500

University of Florida
Special focus: General
Location: Gainesville, FL
Degree granted: Master's Degree
Phone: 352-265-7955
E-mail: cathleen.burdette@medicine.ufl.edu
Website: http://medinfo.ufl.edu/pa/
Supplemental application: Yes
Number of students accepted into program each year: 60
Average GPA: 3.6
GRE: Yes
Length of program: 24 months
Uses CASPA: Yes
Tuition Cost: $55,940

Georgia PA Programs

Emory University School of Medicine
Special focus: Primary Care
Location: Atlanta, GA
Degree granted: Master's Degree
Phone: 404-727-7825
E-mail: emory-pa-admit@learnlink.emory.edu
Website: http://www.emorypa.org/
Supplemental application: Yes, $30 fee
Number of students accepted into program each year: 50
Average GPA: 3.4
GRE: Yes
Length of program: 28 month
Uses CASPA: Yes
Tuition Cost: $50,400

Medical College of Georgia
Special focus: General
Location: Augusta, GA
Degree granted: Master's Degree
Phone: 706-721-2725
E-mail: wpaschal@mcg.edu
Website: http://www.mcg.edu/sah/phyasst/
Supplemental application: Yes
Number of students accepted into program each year: 40
Average GPA: 3.4
GRE: Yes
Length of program: 27 months
Uses CASPA: No
Tuition Cost: $27,000 (in-state), $54,504 (out-of-state)

Mercer University College of Pharmacy and Health Sciences
Special focus: Primary Care
Location: Atlanta, GA
Degree granted: Master's Degree
Phone: 678-547-6232
E-mail: paprogram@mercer.edu
Website: http://cophs.mercer.edu/pa.htm
Supplemental application: No
Number of students accepted into program each year: 26
Average GPA: >3.0
GRE: Yes
Length of program: 28 months
Uses CASPA: Yes
Tuition Cost: $40,716

South University
Special focus: General
Location: Savannah, GA
Degree granted: Master's Degree
Phone: 912-201-8025
E-mail: paprogram@southuniversity.edu
Website: http://www.southuniversity.edu/campus/PhysicianAssistant/
index.asp?siteID=
Supplemental application: No
Number of students accepted into program each year: 70
Average GPA: >2.6
GRE: Yes
Length of program: 27 months
Uses CASPA: Yes
Tuition Cost: $55,755

Iowa PA Programs

Des Moines University
Special focus: General
Location: Des Moines, IA
Degree granted: Master's Degree
Phone: 515-271-7875
E-mail: paadmit@dmu.edu
Website: http://www.dmu.edu/pa/
Supplemental application: No
Number of students accepted into program each year: 44
Average GPA: 3.5
GRE: Yes
Length of program: 25 months
Uses CASPA: Yes
Tuition Cost: $46,380

University of Iowa
Special focus: General
Location: Iowa City, IA
Degree granted: Master's Degree
Phone: 319-335-8922
E-mail: paprogram@uiowa.edu
Website: http://paprogram.medicine.uiowa.edu/
Supplemental application: No
Number of students accepted into program each year: 25
Average GPA: 3.5
GRE: Yes
Length of program: 25 months
Uses CASPA: Yes
Tuition Cost: $17,124 (in-state), $49,836 (out-of-state)

Idaho PA Programs

Idaho State University
Special focus: General
Location: Pocatello, ID and Boise, ID
Degree granted: Master's Degree
Phone: 208-282-4726
E-mail: pa@isu.edu
Website: http://www.isu.edu/PAprog/index.shtml
Supplemental application: Yes
Number of students accepted into program each year: 30 (Pocatello), and 20 (Boise)
Average GPA: 3.6
GRE: Yes
Length of program: 24 months
Uses CASPA: Yes
Tuition Cost: $15,540 (in-state), $41,340 (out-of-state)

Illinois PA Programs

John H. Stroger, Jr. Hospital of Cook County /Malcolm X College
Special focus: General
Location: Chicago, IL
Degree granted: Certificate
Phone: 312-850-7159
E-mail: PAProgram@ccc.edu
Website: http://malcolmx.ccc.edu/aas/physicianAssist/default.asp
Supplemental application: Yes
Number of students accepted into program each year: 30
Average GPA: N/A
GRE: No
Length of program: 25 months
Uses CASPA: No
Tuition Cost: $5,616 (in-county), $22,776 (out-of-county)

Midwestern University
Special focus: General
Location: Downers Grove, IL
Degree granted: Master's Degree
Phone: 800-458-6253
E-mail: admissil@midwestern.edu
Website: http://www.midwestern.edu/il-pa/
Supplemental application: No
Number of students accepted into program each year: 84
Average GPA: >2.75
GRE: Yes
Length of program: 27 months
Uses CASPA: Yes
Tuition Cost: $57,856

Rosalind Franklin University of Medicine and Science
Special focus: General
Location: North Chicago, IL
Degree granted: Master's Degree
Phone: 847-589-8686
E-mail: pa.admissions@rosalindfranklin.edu
Website: http://www.rosalindfranklin.edu/srhs/passt/MS1.cfm
Supplemental application: Yes, $25 fee
Number of students accepted into program each year: 55
Average GPA: >3.0
GRE: Yes
Length of program: 24 months
Uses CASPA: Yes
Tuition Cost: $41,428

Southern Illinois University at Carbondale
Special focus: General
Location: Carbondale, IL
Degree granted: Master's Degree
Phone: 618-453-5527
E-mail: pa_advisement@siumed.edu
Website: http://www.siu.edu/~sah/pa.html
Supplemental application: Yes, $45 fee
Number of students accepted into program each year: 24
Average GPA: >2.8
GRE: Yes
Length of program: 26 months
Uses CASPA: No
Tuition Cost: $40,000 (in-state), $80,000 (out-of-state)

Indiana PA Programs

Butler University/Clarian Health
Special focus: General
Location: Indianapolis, IN
Degree granted: Master's Degree
Phone: 317-940-9969
E-mail: dpearson@butler.edu
Website: http://www.butler.edu/cophs/?pg=2077&parentID=2041
Supplemental application: No
Number of students accepted into program each year: 50
Average GPA: 3.3
GRE: No
Length of program: 36 months
Uses CASPA: Yes
Tuition Cost: $94,920

University of Saint Francis
Special focus: General
Location: Fort Wayne, IN
Degree granted: Master's Degree
Phone: 260-434-3279
E-mail: jcashdollar@sf.edu
Website: http://www.sf.edu/healthscience/pa/index.shtml
Supplemental application: No
Number of students accepted into program each year: 25
Average GPA: >3.0
GRE: Yes
Length of program: 27 months
Uses CASPA: Yes
Tuition Cost: $60,760

Kansas PA Programs

Wichita State University
Special focus: General
Location: Wichita, KS
Degree granted: Master's Degree
Phone: 316-978-3011
E-mail: dee.mcdaniel@wichita.edu
Website: http://webs.wichita.edu/?u=chp_pa&p=/index
Supplemental application: Yes
Number of students accepted into program each year: 42 students
Average GPA: >3.0
GRE: No
Length of program: 26 months
Uses CASPA: Yes
Tuition Cost: $17,028 (in-state), $47,128 (out-of-state)

Kentucky PA Programs

University of Kentucky
Special focus: Primary Care
Location: Lexington, KY
Degree granted: Master's Degree
Phone: 859-323-1100
E-mail: gagair01@e-mail.uky.edu
Website: http://www.mc.uky.edu/PA/
Supplemental application: Yes
Number of students accepted into program each year: 40
Average GPA: 3.4
GRE: Yes
Length of program: 30 months
Uses CASPA: No
Tuition Cost: $31,000

Louisiana PA Programs

Louisiana State University Health Sciences Center
Special focus: Primary Care
Location: Shreveport, LA
Degree granted: Bachelor's Degree
Phone: 318-813-2920
E-mail: kmeyer1@lsuhsc.edu
Website: http://www.medcom.lsuhsc-s.edu/cfide/AlliedHealth/
ACD_physician_assistant.cfm
Supplemental application: Yes
Number of students accepted into program each year: 36
Average GPA: 3.6
GRE: No
Length of program: 27 months
Uses CASPA: No
Tuition Cost: $12,000

Our Lady of the Lake College
Special focus: General
Location: Baton Rouge, LA
Degree granted: Master's Degree
Phone: 225-214-6988
E-mail: egrant@ololcollege.edu
Website: http://www.ololcollege.edu/physician_asst.html
Supplemental application: No
Number of students accepted into program each year: 30
Average GPA: 3.3
GRE: Yes
Length of program: 28 months
Uses CASPA: Yes
Tuition Cost: $22,880

Massachusetts PA Programs

Massachusetts College of Pharmacy and Health Sciences
Special focus: General
Location: Boston, MA
Degree granted: Master's Degree
Phone: 617-732-2918
E-mail: admissions@bos.mcphs.edu
Website: http://www.mcphs.edu/academics/programs/physician_assistant_studies/index.html
Supplemental application: Yes, $40 fee
Number of students accepted into program each year: 30
Average GPA: 3.5
GRE: No
Length of program: 30 months
Uses CASPA: Yes
Tuition Cost: $66,000

Northeastern University
Special focus: General
Location: Boston, MA
Degree granted: Master's Degree
Phone: 617-373-3195
E-mail: paprogram@neu.edu
Website: http://marcom1.neu.edu/bouve/programs/mphysassist.html
Supplemental application: Yes, $50 fee
Number of students accepted into program each year: 34
Average GPA: >3.0
GRE: No
Length of program: 24 months
Uses CASPA: No
Tuition Cost: $46,920

Springfield College/Baystate Health System
Special focus: Primary Care
Location: Springfield, MA
Degree granted: Bachelor's Degree, and Master's Degree
Phone: 800-343-1257
E-mail: glabelle@spfldcol.edu
Website: http://www.spfldcol.edu/homepage/hsrs.nsf/DCC0DBBEC0FAE5B
5852571B2004F2443/22F1A39E7A04388A852571C500625B0A?OpenDocument
Supplemental application: No
Number of students accepted into program each year: 30
Average GPA: >3.0
GRE: No
Length of program: 27 months
Uses CASPA: Yes
Tuition Cost: N/A

Maryland PA Programs

Anne Arundel Community College
Special focus: General
Location: Arnold, MD
Degree granted: Certificate, Master's Degree option
Phone: 410-777-7310
E-mail: laramos@aacc.edu
Website: http://www.aacc.edu/physassist/
Supplemental application: Yes, $25 fee
Number of students accepted into program each year: 40
Average GPA: 3.4
GRE: No
Length of program: 25 months
Uses CASPA: Yes
Tuition Cost: $19,024 (in-state), $39.830 (out-of-state)

Towson University - CCBC Essex
Special focus: General
Location: Baltimore, MD
Degree granted: Master's Degree
Phone: 410-780-6159
E-mail: sshaw@ccbcmd.edu
Website: http://wwwnew.towson.edu/chp/pa/
Supplemental application: Yes
Number of students accepted into program each year: 35
Average GPA: >3.0
GRE: No
Length of program: 26 months
Uses CASPA: Yes
Tuition Cost: $18,861 (in-state), $38,616 (out-of-state)

University of Maryland-Eastern Shore
Special focus: General
Location: Princess Anne, MD
Degree granted: Bachelor's Degree
Phone: 410-651-7584
E-mail: pa@mail.umes.edu
Website: http://www.umes.edu/Academic/SHP/PA/
Supplemental application: Yes
Number of students accepted into program each year: 35
Average GPA: >3.0
GRE: No
Length of program: 4 years
Uses CASPA: No
Tuition Cost: $37,860 (in-state), $73,038 (out-of-state)

Maine PA Programs

The University of New England
Special focus: Primary Care
Location: Biddeford, ME
Degree granted: Master's Degree
Phone: 207-221-4529
E-mail: bdoyle@une.edu
Website: http://www.une.edu/chp/pa/
Supplemental application: No
Number of students accepted into program each year: N/A
Average GPA: N/A
GRE: No
Length of program: 24 months
Uses CASPA: Yes
Tuition Cost: $58,260

Michigan PA Programs

Central Michigan University
Special focus: General
Location: Mount Pleasant, MI
Degree granted: Master's Degree
Phone: 989-774-2478
E-mail: chpadmit@cmich.edu
Website: http://www.chp.cmich.edu/pa/default.htm
Supplemental application: Yes
Number of students accepted into program each year: 45
Average GPA: 3.4
GRE: Yes
Length of program: 27 months
Uses CASPA: Yes
Tuition Cost: $46,560 (in-state), $86,280 (out-of-state)

Grand Valley State University
Special focus: General
Location: Grand Rapids, MI
Degree granted: Master's Degree
Phone: 616-331-3356
E-mail: pas@gvsu.edu
Website: http://www.gvsu.edu/pa/
Supplemental application: Yes
Number of students accepted into program each year: N/A
Average GPA: 3.2
GRE: No
Length of program: 32 months
Uses CASPA: No
Tuition Cost: $37,060 (in-state), $62,675 (out-of-state)

University of Detroit Mercy
Special focus: Primary Care
Location: Detroit, MI
Degree granted: Master's Degree
Phone: 313-993-2474
E-mail: chpgrad@udmercy.edu
Website: http://healthprofessions.udmercy.edu/paprogram/
Supplemental application: Yes
Number of students accepted into program each year: 30-40
Average GPA: 3.3
GRE: Yes
Length of program: 24 months or 36 months
Uses CASPA: Yes
Tuition Cost: $60,120

Wayne State University
Special focus: General
Location: Detroit, MI
Degree granted: Master's Degree
Phone: 313-577-1368
E-mail: ac2605@wayne.edu
Website: http://www.pa.cphs.wayne.edu/default.htm
Supplemental application: Yes
Number of students accepted into program each year: 50
Average GPA: >3.0
GRE: Yes
Length of program: N/A
Uses CASPA: Yes
Tuition Cost: $21,708 (in-state), $48,000 (out-of-state)

Western Michigan University
Special focus: Primary Care
Location: Kalamazoo, MI
Degree granted: Master's Degree
Phone: 269-387-5311
E-mail: feen@wmich.edu
Website: http://www.wmich.edu/hhs/pa/
Supplemental application: No
Number of students accepted into program each year: 40
Average GPA: >3.0
GRE: No
Length of program: 24 months
Uses CASPA: Yes
Tuition Cost: $32,747 (in-state), $69,350 (out-of-state)

Minnesota PA Programs

Augsburg College
Special focus: General
Location: Minneapolis, MN
Degree granted: Master's Degree
Phone: 612-330-1399
E-mail: paprog@augsburg.edu
Website: http://www.augsburg.edu/pa/
Supplemental application: Yes
Number of students accepted into program each year: 28
Average GPA: >3.0
GRE: No
Length of program: 36 months
Uses CASPA: Yes
Tuition Cost: $62,500

Missouri PA Programs

Missouri State University
Special focus: Primary Care
Location: Springfield, MO
Degree granted: Master's Degree
Phone: 417-836-6151
E-mail: physicianasststudies@smsu.edu
Website: http://www.missouristate.edu/pas/default.htm
Supplemental application: No
Number of students accepted into program each year: 24
Average GPA: 3.4
GRE: Yes
Length of program: 24 months
Uses CASPA: Yes
Tuition Cost: $17,098 (in-state), $33,366 (out-of-state)

Saint Louis University
Special focus: General
Location: St. Louis, MO
Degree granted: Master's Degree
Phone: 314-977-8521
E-mail: paprog@slu.edu
Website: http://www.slu.edu/x2348.xml
Supplemental application: Yes, $25 fee
Number of students accepted into program each year: 34
Average GPA: >3.0
GRE: No
Length of program: 27 months
Uses CASPA: Yes
Tuition Cost: $60,465

Montana PA Programs

Rocky Mountain College
Special focus: General
Location: Billings, MT
Degree granted: Master's Degree
Phone: 406-657-1190
E-mail: pa@rocky.edu
Website: http://www.rocky.edu/?type=schoolOfAlliedHealth
Supplemental application: Yes
Number of students accepted into program each year: 28
Average GPA: >3.0
GRE: Yes
Length of program: 26 months
Uses CASPA: Yes
Tuition Cost: $56,000

North Carolina PA Programs

Duke University Medical Center
Special focus: General
Location: Durham, NC
Degree granted: Master's Degree
Phone: 919-681-3161
E-mail: paadmission@mc.duke.edu
Website: http://pa.mc.duke.edu/
Supplemental application: Yes
Number of students accepted into program each year: 60
Average GPA: 3.3
GRE: Yes
Length of program: 24 months
Uses CASPA: Yes
Tuition Cost: $54,064

East Carolina University
Special focus: Primary Care
Location: Greenville, NC
Degree granted: Master's Degree
Phone: 252-744-1100
E-mail: pastudies@mail.ecu.edu
Website: http://www.ecu.edu/pa/
Supplemental application: Yes, $60 fee
Number of students accepted into program each year: 30
Average GPA: >3.0
GRE: Yes
Length of program: 27 months
Uses CASPA: Yes
Tuition Cost: $17,018 (in-state), $55,414 (out-of-state)

Methodist University
Special focus: General
Location: Fayetteville, NC
Degree granted: Master's Degree
Phone: 910-630-7495
E-mail: paprog@methodist.edu
Website: http://www.methodist.edu/paprogram/index.htm
Supplemental application: No
Number of students accepted into program each year: 34
Average GPA: >3.0
GRE: Yes
Length of program: 27 months
Uses CASPA: Yes
Tuition Cost: $56,120

Wake Forest University
Special focus: General
Location: Winston-Salem, NC
Degree granted: Master's Degree
Phone: 336-716-4356
E-mail: kscales@wfubmc.edu
Website: http://www1.wfubmc.edu/PAprogram/
Supplemental application: No
Number of students accepted into program each year: 48
Average GPA: 3.3
GRE: Yes
Length of program: 24 months
Uses CASPA: Yes
Tuition Cost: $43,310

North Dakota PA Programs

University of North Dakota School of Medicine and Health Sciences
Special focus: Primary Care
Location: Grand Forks, ND
Degree granted: Master's Degree
Phone: 701-777-2344
E-mail: painfo@medicine.nodak.edu
Website: http://www.med.und.nodak.edu/physicianassistant/
Supplemental application: Yes, $35 fee
Number of students accepted into program each year: 70
Average GPA: >2.75
GRE: No
Length of program: 24 months
Uses CASPA: No
Tuition Cost: $30,000

Nebraska PA Programs

Union College
Special focus: Primary Care
Location: Lincoln, NE
Degree granted: Master's Degree
Phone: 402-486-2527
E-mail: paprog@ucollege.edu
Website: http://www.ucollege.edu/ucscripts/public/template/
default.asp?DivID=1&pgID=301
Supplemental application: No
Number of students accepted into program each year: 25
Average GPA: 3.3
GRE: No
Length of program: 32 months
Uses CASPA: Yes
Tuition Cost: $82,000

University of Nebraska Medical Center
Special focus: General
Location: Omaha, NE
Degree granted: Master's Degree
Phone: 402-559-9495
E-mail: dklandon@unmc.edu
Website: http://www.unmc.edu/dept/alliedhealth/pa/
Supplemental application: Yes
Number of students accepted into program each year: 40
Average GPA: 3.75
GRE: Yes
Length of program: 28 months
Uses CASPA: Yes
Tuition Cost: $27,552 (in-state), $74,292 (out-of-state)

New Hampshire PA Programs

Massachusetts College of Pharmacy and Health Sciences-Manchester
Special focus: General
Location: Manchester, NH
Degree granted: Master's Degree
Phone: 603-314-1730
E-mail: admissions@man.mcphs.edu
Website: http://www.mcphs.edu/academics/programs/physician%5Fassistant%5F
studies/PA%5F24%5FMan/
Supplemental application: Yes
Number of students accepted into program each year: 40
Average GPA: 3.4
GRE: No
Length of program: 24 months
Uses CASPA: Yes
Tuition Cost: $66,000

New Jersey PA Programs

Seton Hall University
Special focus: General
Location: South Orange, NJ
Degree granted: Master's Degree
Phone: 973-275-2596
E-mail: gradmeded@shu.edu
Website: http://www.shu.edu/academics/gradmeded/ms-physician-assistant/index.cfm
Supplemental application: Yes
Number of students accepted into program each year: N/A
Average GPA: >3.0
GRE: Yes
Length of program: 36 months
Uses CASPA: No
Tuition Cost: $79,296

University of Medicine and Dentistry of New Jersey
Special focus: Primary Care
Location: Piscataway, NJ
Degree granted: Master's Degree, optional Bachelor's Degree
Phone: 732-235-4445
E-mail: pa-info@umdnj.edu
Website: http://shrp.umdnj.edu/programs/paweb/index.html
Supplemental application: Yes
Number of students accepted into program each year: 50-60
Average GPA: >3.0
GRE: No
Length of program: 36 months
Uses CASPA: No
Tuition Cost: $52,152 (in-state), $78,228 (out-of-state)

New Mexico PA Programs

The University of New Mexico School of Medicine
Special focus: General
Location: Albuquerque, NM
Degree granted: Bachelor's Degree
Phone: 505-272-9678
E-mail: paprogram@salud.unm.edu
Website: http://hsc.unm.edu/som/fcm/pap/
Supplemental application: Yes
Number of students accepted into program each year: 15
Average GPA: 3.5
GRE: No
Length of program: 25 months
Uses CASPA: Yes
Tuition Cost: $15,030 (in-state), $36,292 (out-of-state)

University of St. Francis
Special focus: General
Location: Albuquerque, NM
Degree granted: Master's Degree
Phone: 888-446-4657
E-mail: pa@stfrancis.edu
Website: http://www.stfrancis.edu/conah/pa/
Supplemental application: No
Number of students accepted into program each year: 30
Average GPA: >2.75
GRE: Yes
Length of program: 27 months
Uses CASPA: Yes
Tuition Cost: $50,742

Nevada PA Programs

Touro University-Nevada
Special focus: General
Location: Henderson, NV
Degree granted: Master's Degree
Phone: 702-777-1750
E-mail: admissionsnv@touro.edu
Website: http://www.tu.edu/departments.php?id=72
Supplemental application: Yes, $50 fee
Number of students accepted into program each year: 50
Average GPA: >2.7
GRE: No
Length of program: 30 months
Uses CASPA: Yes
Tuition Cost: $55,000

New York PA Programs

Albany Medical College
Special focus: General
Location: Albany, NY
Degree granted: Master's Degree
Phone: 518-262-5251
E-mail: greenr@mail.amc.edu
Website: http://www.amc.edu/Academic/PhysicianAssistant/
Supplemental application: Yes, $50 fee
Number of students accepted into program each year: 30-35
Average GPA: 3.36
GRE: Yes
Length of program: 28 months
Uses CASPA: Yes
Tuition Cost: $42,000

CUNY York College
Special focus: General
Location: Jamaica, NY
Degree granted: Bachelor's Degree
Phone: 718-262-2823
E-mail: paprogram@york.cuny.edu
Website: http://med.cuny.edu/pap/
Supplemental application: Yes
Number of students accepted into program each year: 30
Average GPA: 2.7
GRE: No
Length of program: 28 months
Uses CASPA: No
Tuition Cost: $12,000 (in-state), $17,000 (out-of-state)

D'Youville College
Special focus: General
Location: Buffalo, NY
Degree granted: Master's Degree, and Bachelor's Degree (BS to MS program)
Phone: 716-881-7713
E-mail: paprogram@dyc.edu
Website: http://www.dyc.edu/academics/physician_assistant/index.asp
Supplemental application: Yes
Number of students accepted into program each year: N/A
Average GPA: >3.0
GRE: No
Length of program: 5 years
Uses CASPA: No
Tuition Cost: $88,000

Daemen College
Special focus: General
Location: Amherst, NY
Degree granted: Master's Degree, and Bachelor's option
Phone: 716- 839-8383
E-mail: mmoore@daemen.edu
Website: http://www.daemen.edu/academics/physician_assistant/
Supplemental application: No
Number of students accepted into program each year: N/A
Average GPA: >3.0
GRE: No
Length of program: 3 years (Master's), and 5 years (Bachelor's)
Uses CASPA: Yes
Tuition Cost: $88,960

Hofstra University
Special focus: General
Location: Hempstead, NY
Degree granted: Master's Degree
Phone: 516-463-4074
E-mail: paprogram@hofstra.edu
Website: http://www.hofstra.edu/Academics/Colleges/HCLAS/PAP/
Supplemental application: Yes
Number of students accepted into program each year: 30
Average GPA: >3.0
GRE: No
Length of program: 24 months
Uses CASPA: No
Tuition Cost: $52,890

Le Moyne College
Special focus: General
Location: Syracuse, NY
Degree granted: Master's Degree
Phone: 315-445-4745
E-mail: PhysAssist@lemoyne.edu
Website: http://www.lemoyne.edu/pa/index.htm
Supplemental application: Yes
Number of students accepted into program each year: 35
Average GPA: >3.0
GRE: No
Length of program: 24 months
Uses CASPA: Yes
Tuition Cost: $59,990

Long Island University
Special focus: General
Location: Brooklyn, NY
Degree granted: Bachelor's Degree
Phone: 718-488-1011
E-mail: pastudies@brooklyn.liu.edu
Website: http://www.brooklyn.liu.edu/health/bsphyass.html
Supplemental application: No
Number of students accepted into program each year: N/A
Average GPA: N/A
GRE: No
Length of program: 4 years
Uses CASPA: Yes
Tuition Cost: $51,657

Mercy College
Special focus: Family Medicine
Location: Bronx, NY
Degree granted: Master's Degree, and Bachelor's Degree
Phone: 914-674-7635
E-mail: paprogram@mercynet.edu
Website: http://mercy.edu/acadivisions/healthprofessions/grad/
physician_assistant.cfm
Supplemental application: No
Number of students accepted into program each year: 20
Average GPA: >3.0
GRE: No
Length of program: 27 months
Uses CASPA: Yes
Tuition Cost: $56,700

New York Institute of Technology
Special focus: General
Location: Old Westbury, NY
Degree granted: Master's Degree
Phone: 516-686-3881
E-mail: lherman@nyit.edu
Website: http://iris.nyit.edu/hpbls/pas/
Supplemental application: No
Number of students accepted into program each year: 52
Average GPA: 3.3
GRE: No
Length of program: 30 months
Uses CASPA: Yes
Tuition Cost: $72,422

Pace University-Lenox Hill Hospital
Special focus: General
Location: New York, NY
Degree granted: Master's Degree
Phone: 212-346-1291
E-mail: paprogram@pace.edu
Website: http://appserv.pace.edu/execute/page.cfm?doc_id=6594
Supplemental application: No
Number of students accepted into program each year: 50
Average GPA: >3.0
GRE: No
Length of program: 26 months
Uses CASPA: Yes
Tuition Cost: $65,056

Rochester Institute of Technology
Special focus: General
Location: Rochester, NY
Degree granted: Bachelor's Degree
Phone: 716-475-2978
E-mail: hbmscl@rit.edu
Website: http://www.rit.edu/~676www/physician_assistant.html
Supplemental application: Yes
Number of students accepted into program each year: 25
Average GPA: 3.0
GRE: No
Length of program: 4 years
Uses CASPA: No
Tuition Cost: $36,612

SUNY/Downstate Medical Center
Special focus: Primary Care
Location: Brooklyn, NY
Degree granted: Bachelor's Degree
Phone: 718-270-2325
E-mail: admissions@downstate.edu
Website: http://www.downstate.edu/pa/default.html
Supplemental application: Yes
Number of students accepted into program each year: 33
Average GPA: >2.75
GRE: No
Length of program: 27 months
Uses CASPA: No
Tuition Cost: $26,100 (in-state), $63,660 (out-of-state)

St. John's University
Special focus: General
Location: Fresh Meadows, NY
Degree granted: Bachelor's Degree
Phone: 718-990-8417
E-mail: N/A
Website: http://new.stjohns.edu/academics/undergraduate/pharmacy/programs/pa
Supplemental application: Yes, $50 fee
Number of students accepted into program each year: N/A
Average GPA: >3.0
GRE: No
Length of program: 24 months
Uses CASPA: Yes
Tuition Cost: $66,000

Stony Brook University
Special focus: Primary Care
Location: Stony Brook, NY
Degree granted: Master's Degree
Phone: 631-444-3190
E-mail: paprogram@stonybrook.edu
Website: http://www.hsc.stonybrook.edu/shtm/pa/index.cfm
Supplemental application: No
Number of students accepted into program each year: 40
Average GPA: 3.2
GRE: No
Length of program: 24 months
Uses CASPA: Yes
Tuition Cost: $25,722 (in-state), $37,785 (out-of-state)

Touro College
Special focus: General
Location: Bay Shore, NY
Degree granted: Bachelor's Degree
Phone: 631-665-1600 ext. 254
E-mail: ngraff@touro.edu
Website: http://www.touro.edu/shs/pa.asp
Supplemental application: Yes, $50 fee
Number of students accepted into program each year: 76
Average GPA: >3.0
GRE: No
Length of program: N/A
Uses CASPA: Yes
Tuition Cost: $34,340

Touro College - Manhattan Campus
Special focus: General
Location: New York, NY
Degree granted: Bachelor's Degree and Master's Degree
Phone: 212-463-0400, ext. 792
E-mail: ngraff@touro.edu
Website: http://www.touro.edu/shs/pany/newBS.asp
Supplemental application: Yes
Number of students accepted into program each year: 40
Average GPA: 3.2
GRE: No
Length of program: 32 months (BS to MS)
Uses CASPA: Yes
Tuition Cost: $36,750

Wagner College/Staten Island University Hospital
Special focus: General
Location: Staten Island, NY
Degree granted: Master's Degree, and Bachelor's Degree option
Phone: 718-390-4615
E-mail: kcromeyer@siuh.edu
Website: http://www.wagner.edu/departments/biological_sciences/
PA/physician_assistant_home
Supplemental application: Yes
Number of students accepted into program each year: 20
Average GPA: >2.7
GRE: No
Length of program: Three years
Uses CASPA: No
Tuition Cost: N/A

Weill Cornell Medical College
Special focus: Surgical
Location: New York, NY
Degree granted: Certificate
Phone: 646-962-7277
E-mail: atc2002@med.cornell.edu
Website: http://www.med.cornell.edu/education/programs/phy_ass.html
Supplemental application: Yes, $60 fee
Number of students accepted into program each year: 32
Average GPA: 3.4
GRE: No
Length of program: 26 months
Uses CASPA: Yes
Tuition Cost: $53,877

Ohio PA Programs

Cuyahoga Community College
Special focus: Primary Care
Location: Parma, OH
Degree granted: Master's Degree
Phone: 216-987-5123
E-mail: sharon.luke@tri-c.edu
Website: http://www.tri-c.edu/PA/docs/program.htm
Supplemental application: Yes
Number of students accepted into program each year: 30
Average GPA: >3.0
GRE: Yes
Length of program: 27 months
Uses CASPA: Yes
Tuition Cost: $30,000

Kettering College of Medical Arts
Special focus: General
Location: Kettering, OH
Degree granted: Master's Degree
Phone: 937-296-7238
E-mail: sue.wulff@kcma.edu
Website: http://www.kcma.edu/Academics/PA/index.html
Supplemental application: No
Number of students accepted into program each year: 35-40
Average GPA: >3.0
GRE: No
Length of program: 27 months
Uses CASPA: Yes
Tuition Cost: N/A

Marietta College
Special focus: General
Location: Marietta, OH
Degree granted: Master's Degree
Phone: 740-376-4458
E-mail: paprog@marietta.edu
Website: http://www.marietta.edu/~paprog/
Supplemental application: Yes
Number of students accepted into program each year: 22
Average GPA: >2.8
GRE: Yes
Length of program: 27 months
Uses CASPA: Yes
Tuition Cost: $60,612

The University of Findlay
Special focus: General
Location: Findlay, OH
Degree granted: Bachelor's Degree
Phone: 419-434-4529
E-mail: pentz@findlay.edu
Website: http://www.findlay.edu/academics/colleges/cohp/academicprograms/
undergraduate/PHAS/default.htm
Supplemental application: Yes
Number of students accepted into program each year: 18
Average GPA: 3.4
GRE: No
Length of program: 27 months
Uses CASPA: Yes
Tuition Cost: $57,595

University of Toledo
Special focus: General
Location: Toledo, OH
Degree granted: Master's Degree
Phone: 419-383-5408
E-mail: tlangenderfe@mco.edu
Website: http://hsc.utoledo.edu/allh/pa/index.html
Supplemental application: Yes
Number of students accepted into program each year: 30
Average GPA: >3.0
GRE: No
Length of program: 27 month
Uses CASPA: Yes
Tuition Cost: $29,484 (in-state), $55,920 (out-of-state)

Oklahoma PA Programs

University of Oklahoma
Special focus: General
Location: Oklahoma City, OK
Degree granted: Master's Degree
Phone: 405-271-2058
E-mail: lillie-neal@ouhsc.edu
Website: http://www.okpa.org/Default.aspx?alias=www.okpa.org/paprogram
Supplemental application: Yes
Number of students accepted into program each year: 50
Average GPA: 3.6
GRE: Yes
Length of program: 30 months
Uses CASPA: No
Tuition Cost: $9,600 (in-state), $12,579 (out-of-state)

University of Oklahoma-Tulsa
Special focus: General
Location: Tulsa, OK
Degree granted: Master's Degree
Phone: 918-619-4760
E-mail: leslie-wallace@ouhsc.edu
Website: http://tulsa.ou.edu/pa/index.htm
Supplemental application: Yes
Number of students accepted into program each year: 20-24
Average GPA: 3.5
GRE: Yes
Length of program: 30 months
Uses CASPA: No
Tuition Cost: $17,010 (in-state), $43,260 (out-of-state)

Oregon PA Programs

Oregon Health Sciences University
Special focus: Primary Care
Location: Portland, OR
Degree granted: Master's Degree
Phone: 503-494-1484
E-mail: paprgm@ohsu.edu
Website: http://www.ohsu.edu/pa/
Supplemental application: Yes
Number of students accepted into program each year: 32
Average GPA: 3.4
GRE: Yes
Length of program: 26 months
Uses CASPA: Yes
Tuition Cost: $59,535

Pacific University
Special focus: Primary Care
Location: Forest Grove, OR
Degree granted: Master's Degree
Phone: 503-352-2898
E-mail: pa@pacificu.edu
Website: http://www.pacificu.edu/pa/
Supplemental application: Yes
Number of students accepted into program each year: 42
Average GPA: 3.4
GRE: No
Length of program: 28 months
Uses CASPA: Yes
Tuition Cost: $49,524

Pennsylvania PA Programs

Arcadia University
Special focus: General
Location: Glenside, PA
Degree granted: Master's Degree
Phone: 215-572-2082
E-mail: daysc@arcadia.edu
Website: http://www.arcadia.edu/academic/default.aspx?pid=425
Supplemental application: No
Number of students accepted into program each year: 49
Average GPA: >3.2
GRE: Yes
Length of program: 24 months, or 36 months
Uses CASPA: Yes
Tuition Cost: $56,400

Chatham College
Special focus: Primary Care
Location: Pittsburgh, PA
Degree granted: Master's Degree
Phone: 412-365-1412
E-mail: admissions@chatham.edu
Website: http://www.chatham.edu/departments/healthmgmt/graduate/pa/index.cfm
Supplemental application: No
Number of students accepted into program each year: 50
Average GPA: >3.0
GRE: No
Length of program: 24 months
Uses CASPA: Yes
Tuition Cost: $62,340

DeSales University
Special focus: Primary Care
Location: Center Valley, PA
Degree granted: Master's Degree
Phone: 610-282-1100 ext. 1415
E-mail: Linda.Schroeder@desales.edu
Website: http://www.desales.edu/default.aspx?pageid=331
Supplemental application: Yes
Number of students accepted into program each year: 40
Average GPA: 3.5
GRE: Yes
Length of program: 24 months
Uses CASPA: Yes
Tuition Cost: N/A

Drexel University Hahnemann
Special focus: General
Location: Philadelphia, PA
Degree granted: Master's Degree
Phone: 215-762-8966
E-mail: js64@drexel.edu
Website: http://www.drexel.edu/cnhp/physician_assistant/about.asp
Supplemental application: Yes
Number of students accepted into program each year: 75
Average GPA: 3.2
GRE: No
Length of program: 27 months
Uses CASPA: Yes
Tuition Cost: $58,485

Duquesne University
Special focus: General
Location: Pittsburgh, PA
Degree granted: Bachelor's Degree, and Master's Degree
Phone: 800-456-5914
E-mail: calhoun@duq.edu
Website: http://www.healthsciences.duq.edu/pa/pahome.html
Supplemental application: Yes
Number of students accepted into program each year: N/A
Average GPA: >3.0
GRE: No
Length of program: Five years (BS to MS)
Uses CASPA: No
Tuition Cost: N/A

Gannon University
Special focus: General
Location: Erie, PA
Degree granted: Bachelor's Degree, and Master's Degree
Phone: 814-871-7474
E-mail: gillespi002@gannon.edu
Website: http://www.gannon.edu/departmental/pa/default.asp
Supplemental application: Yes
Number of students accepted into program each year: 40
Average GPA: >3.2
GRE: No
Length of program: Five years (BS), and 29 months (MS)
Uses CASPA: No
Tuition Cost: $83,460

Kings College
Special focus: General
Location: Wilkes-Barre, PA
Degree granted: Bachelor's Degree, and Master's Degree
Phone: 570-208-5853
E-mail: suzannesedon@kings.edu
Website: http://departments.kings.edu/paprog/
Supplemental application: No
Number of students accepted into program each year: 44
Average GPA: >3.0
GRE: No
Length of program: Five years (BS to MS), and 24 months (MS)
Uses CASPA: Yes
Tuition Cost: N/A

Lock Haven University of Pennsylvania
Special focus: General
Location: Lock Haven, PA
Degree granted: Master's Degree
Phone: 570-893-2541
E-mail: weisenha@lhup.edu
Website: http://gradprograms.lhup.edu/pa/
Supplemental application: No
Number of students accepted into program each year: N/A
Average GPA: >3.0
GRE: Yes
Length of program: 24 months
Uses CASPA: Yes
Tuition Cost: $28,278 (in-state), $42,184 (out-of-state)

Marywood University
Special focus: General, with option to specialize
Location: Scranton, PA
Degree granted: Master's Degree
Phone: 570-348-6298
E-mail: paprogram@marywood.edu
Website: http://www.marywood.edu/departments/pa_program/program.stm
Supplemental application: No
Number of students accepted into program each year: 30-45
Average GPA: 3.0
GRE: No
Length of program: 27 months
Uses CASPA: Yes
Tuition Cost: $53,515

Pennsylvania College of Optometry
Special focus: General
Location: Elkins Park, PA
Degree granted: Master's Degree
Phone: 215-780-1515
E-mail: pa@pco.edu
Website: http://www.pco.edu/pa/pa_whatis.htm
Supplemental application: No
Number of students accepted into program each year: 20
Average GPA: 3.4
GRE: Yes
Length of program: 25 months
Uses CASPA: Yes
Tuition Cost: $50,900

Pennsylvania College of Technology
Special focus: General
Location: Williamsport, PA
Degree granted: Bachelor's Degree
Phone: 570-327-4779
E-mail: pa@pct.edu
Website: http://www.pct.edu/schools/hs/bpa/
Supplemental application: Yes
Number of students accepted into program each year: 30
Average GPA: >3.0
GRE: No
Length of program: 24 months
Uses CASPA: No
Tuition Cost: $57,000 (in-state), $71,592 (out-of-state)

Philadelphia College of Osteopathic Medicine
Special focus: Osteopathic
Location: Philadelphia, PA
Degree granted: Master's Degree
Phone: 215-871-6700
E-mail: admissions@pcom.edu
Website: http://www.pcom.edu/Academic_Programs/aca_pa/
Degree_Programs_Physician_Assi/degree_programs_physician_assi.html
Supplemental application: No
Number of students accepted into program each year: N/A
Average GPA: >2.8
GRE: No
Length of program: 26 months
Uses CASPA: Yes
Tuition Cost: $ 50,534

Philadelphia University
Special focus: General
Location: Philadelphia, PA
Degree granted: Master's Degree
Phone: 215-951-2908
E-mail: rackoverm@PhilaU.edu
Website: http://www.philau.edu/paprogram/
Supplemental application: No
Number of students accepted into program each year: 35
Average GPA: >3.0
GRE: Yes
Length of program: 25 months
Uses CASPA: Yes
Tuition Cost: $58,506

Saint Francis University
Special focus: General
Location: Loretto, PA
Degree granted: Master's Degree, and Bachelor's option
Phone: 814-472-3020
E-mail: pa@francis.edu
Website: http://www.saintfrancisuniversity.edu/MPAShome.htm
Supplemental application: No
Number of students accepted into program each year: 55-60
Average GPA: >3.0
GRE: No
Length of program: 24 months (MS), or five years (BS to MS)
Uses CASPA: Yes
Tuition Cost: $63,102

Seton Hill University
Special focus: General
Location: Greensburg, PA
Degree granted: Master's Degree, and Bachelor's option
Phone: 724-838-4283
E-mail: admit@setonhill.edu
Website: http://www.setonhill.edu/o/index.cfm?PID=24
Supplemental application: No
Number of students accepted into program each year: 26
Average GPA: >3.0
GRE: No
Length of program: 29 months (MS), or five years (BS to MS)
Uses CASPA: Yes
Tuition Cost: $68,805

South Carolina PA Programs

Medical University of South Carolina
Special focus: General
Location: Charleston, SC
Degree granted: Master's Degree
Phone: 843-792-1913
E-mail: rodgersm@musc.edu
Website: http://www.musc.edu/chp/pa/
Supplemental application: Yes
Number of students accepted into program each year: 60
Average GPA: >3.0
GRE: Yes
Length of program: 27 months
Uses CASPA: No
Tuition Cost: $39,802 (in-state), $79,359 (out-of-state)

South Dakota PA Programs

University of South Dakota
Special focus: General
Location: Vermillion, SD
Degree granted: Master's Degree
Phone: 605-677-5128
E-mail: usdpa@usd.edu
Website: http://www.usd.edu/med/pa/
Supplemental application: Yes, $35 fee
Number of students accepted into program each year: 20
Average GPA: >3.0
GRE: No
Length of program: 28 months
Uses CASPA: Yes
Tuition Cost: $13,026 (in-state), $38,407 (out-of-state)

Tennessee PA Programs

South College
Special focus: General
Location: Knoxville, TN
Degree granted: Master's Degree
Phone: 865-251-1800
E-mail: pa_program@southcollegetn.edu
Website: http://www.southcollegetn.edu/masters/physician-assistant/
Supplemental application: Yes
Number of students accepted into program each year: N/A
Average GPA: 3.0
GRE: Yes
Length of program: 27 months
Uses CASPA: No
Tuition Cost: $55,800

Trevecca Nazarene University
Special focus: General
Location: Nashville, TN
Degree granted: Master's Degree
Phone: 615-248-1225
E-mail: admissions_pa@trevecca.edu
Website: http://www.trevecca.edu/pa/
Supplemental application: No
Number of students accepted into program each year: 40
Average GPA: >3.25
GRE: Yes
Length of program: 27 months
Uses CASPA: Yes
Tuition Cost: $63,916

Bethel College
Special focus: General
Location: McKenzie, TN
Degree granted: Master's Degree
Phone: (731) 352-4247
E-mail: atwills@bethel-college.edu
Website: http://www.bethel-college.edu/bethelpa/index.htm
Supplemental application: Yes
Number of students accepted into program each year: N/A
Average GPA: N/A
GRE: Yes
Length of program: 27 months
Uses CASPA: No
Tuition Cost: N/A
(Note: Currently not accredited by ARC-PA, although actively seeking accreditation)

Texas PA Programs

Baylor College of Medicine
Special focus: General
Location: Houston, TX
Degree granted: Master's Degree
Phone: 713-798-4619
E-mail: melodym@bcm.tmc.edu
Website: http://www.bcm.edu/pap/
Supplemental application: Yes
Number of students accepted into program each year: 35
Average GPA: 3.5
GRE: Yes
Length of program: 30 months
Uses CASPA: Yes
Tuition Cost: $35,000

Texas Tech University Health Sciences Center
Special focus: General
Location: Midland, TX
Degree granted: Master's Degree
Phone: 915-620-9905
E-mail: allied.health@ttuhsc.edu
Website: http://www.ttuhsc.edu/sah/mpa/
Supplemental application: Yes
Number of students accepted into program each year: 65
Average GPA: >3.2
GRE: No
Length of program: 27 months
Uses CASPA: Yes
Tuition Cost: $19,131 (in-state), or $44,151 (out-of-state)

The University of Texas - Pan American
Special focus: General
Location: Edinburg, TX
Degree granted: Bachelor's Degree
Phone: 956-381-2298
E-mail: N/A
Website: http://www.utpa.edu/dept/pasp/
Supplemental application: Yes
Number of students accepted into program each year: 25-40
Average GPA: >3.3
GRE: No
Length of program: N/A
Uses CASPA: No
Tuition Cost: $11,368

The University of Texas Health Science Center at San Antonio
Special focus: General
Location: San Antonio, TX
Degree granted: Master's Degree
Phone: 210-567-2660
E-mail: pastudies@uthscsa.edu
Website: http://www.uthscsa.edu/sah/pastudies/
Supplemental application: Yes
Number of students accepted into program each year: 24
Average GPA: >3.0
GRE: No
Length of program: 33 months
Uses CASPA: Yes
Tuition Cost: $18,755

The University of Texas Medical Branch
Special focus: General
Location: Galveston, TX
Degree granted: Master's Degree
Phone: 409-772-3046
E-mail: rrahr@utmb.edu
Website: http://www.sahs.utmb.edu/pas/
Supplemental application: Yes
Number of students accepted into program each year: 40-45
Average GPA: 3.6
GRE: Yes
Length of program: 24 months
Uses CASPA: Yes
Tuition Cost: $19,225 (in-state), $49,527 (out-of-state)

University of North Texas
Special focus: Osteopathic, Primary Care
Location: Fort Worth, TX
Degree granted: Master's Degree
Phone: 817-735-2204
E-mail: PAAdmissions@hsc.unt.edu
Website: http://www.hsc.unt.edu/education/pasp/
Supplemental application: Yes
Number of students accepted into program each year: 36
Average GPA: >2.85
GRE: No
Length of program: 34 months
Uses CASPA: Yes
Tuition Cost: $22,457 (in-state), $62,201 (out-of-state)

University of Texas, Southwestern Medical Center at Dallas
Special focus: General
Location: Dallas, TX
Degree granted: Master's Degree
Phone: 214-648-1701
E-mail: isela.perez@utsouthwestern.edu
Website: http://www8.utsouthwestern.edu/utsw/cda/dept48945/files/54102.html
Supplemental application: No
Number of students accepted into program each year: 36
Average GPA: 3.5
GRE: Yes
Length of program: 31 months
Uses CASPA: Yes
Tuition Cost: $12,840 (in-state), $45,960 (out-of-state)

Utah PA Programs

University of Utah
Special focus: Primary Care
Location: Salt Lake City, UT
Degree granted: Master's Degree
Phone: 801-581-7766
E-mail: admissions@upap.utah.edu
Website: http://web.utah.edu/upap/
Supplemental application: No
Number of students accepted into program each year: 36
Average GPA: >3.0
GRE: No
Length of program: 27 months
Uses CASPA: Yes
Tuition Cost: $47,541 (in-state), $70,785 (out-of-state)

Virginia PA Programs

Eastern Virginia Medical School
Special focus: General
Location: Norfolk, VA
Degree granted: Master's Degree
Phone: 757-446-7158
E-mail: paprog@evms.edu
Website: http://www.evms.edu/hlthprof/mpa/
Supplemental application: No
Number of students accepted into program each year: N/A
Average GPA: >3.0
GRE: No
Length of program: 27 months
Uses CASPA: Yes
Tuition Cost: $51,366

James Madison University
Special focus: General
Location: Harrisonburg, VA
Degree granted: Master's Degree
Phone: 540-568-2395
E-mail: paprogram@jmu.edu
Website: http://www.jmu.edu/healthsci/paweb/
Supplemental application: Yes
Number of students accepted into program each year: 25
Average GPA: 3.4
GRE: Yes
Length of program: 28 months
Uses CASPA: Yes
Tuition Cost: $22,645 (in-state), $64,159 (out-of-state)

Jefferson College of Health Sciences
Special focus: Community Medicine
Location: Roanoke, VA
Degree granted: Bachelor's Degree
Phone: 540-985-4016
E-mail: admissions@mail.jchs.edu
Website: http://www.jchs.edu/page.php/prmID/77#69
Supplemental application: No
Number of students accepted into program each year: 40
Average GPA: 3.0
GRE: Yes
Length of program: 24 months
Uses CASPA: Yes
Tuition Cost: $48,860

Shenandoah University
Special focus: General
Location: Winchester, VA
Degree granted: Master's Degree
Phone: 540-542-6208
E-mail: pa@su.edu
Website: http://www.su.edu/pa/
Supplemental application: No
Number of students accepted into program each year: 38
Average GPA: 3.4
GRE: Yes
Length of program: 27 month
Uses CASPA: Yes
Tuition Cost: $53,120

Washington PA Programs

University of Washington
Special focus: Primary Care
Location: Seattle, WA
Degree granted: Certificate, and Master's Degree
Phone: 206-616-4001
E-mail: medex@u.washington.edu
Website: http://www.washington.edu/medicine/som/depts/medex/
Supplemental application: Yes
Number of students accepted into program each year: 93
Average GPA: >2.7
GRE: No
Length of program: N/A
Uses CASPA: Yes
Tuition Cost: $40,560

Wisconsin PA Programs

Marquette University
Special focus: Primary Care
Location: Milwaukee, WI
Degree granted: Master's Degree, and Bachelor's option
Phone: 414-288-5688
E-mail: sandy.dziatkiewicz@marquette.edu
Website: http://www.marquette.edu/chs/pa/index.shtml
Supplemental application: Yes
Number of students accepted into program each year: 50
Average GPA: 3.25
GRE: No
Length of program: 31 months
Uses CASPA: No
Tuition Cost: $78,810

University of Wisconsin-LaCrosse-Gunderson Lutheran Medical Foundation/Mayo School of Health-Related Sciences
Special focus: General
Location: LaCrosse, WI
Degree granted: Master's Degree
Phone: 608-785-8470
E-mail: paprogram@uwlax.edu
Website: http://perth.uwlax.edu/pastudies/
Supplemental application: Yes
Number of students accepted into program each year: 12-14
Average GPA: 3.7
GRE: Yes
Length of program: 24 months
Uses CASPA: Yes
Tuition Cost: $23,160 (in-state), $63,600 (out-of-state)

University of Wisconsin-Madison
Special focus: General
Location: Madison, WI
Degree granted: Bachelor's Degree, Master's Degree (begins 2009)
Phone: 608-263-5620
E-mail: paprogram@mailplus.wisc.edu
Website: http://www.physicianassistant.wisc.edu/
Supplemental application: Yes
Number of students accepted into program each year: 30
Average GPA: 3.0
GRE: No
Length of program: 24 months
Uses CASPA: Yes
Tuition Cost: $21,570 (in-state), $64,320 (out-of-state)

West Virginia PA Programs

Alderson Broaddus College
Special focus: General
Location: Philippi, WV
Degree granted: Master's Degree
Phone: 304-457-6283
E-mail: holt_m@ab.edu
Website: http://www.ab.edu/academics/degrees/physician_assistant_studies
Supplemental application: No
Number of students accepted into program each year: 45
Average GPA: 3.0
GRE: No
Length of program: Three years
Uses CASPA: Yes
Tuition Cost: $75,560

Mountain State University
Special focus: Primary Care
Location: Beckley, WV
Degree granted: Master's Degree, and Bachelor's option
Phone: 304-253-7351
E-mail: dcampbell@mountainstate.edu
Website: http://www.mountainstate.edu/majors/onlinecatalogs/
graduate/programs/PhysiciansAssistant.aspx
Supplemental application: Yes
Number of students accepted into program each year: 25-30
Average GPA: 3.0
GRE: No
Length of program: <48 months
Uses CASPA: No
Tuition Cost: N/A

Uniformed PA Programs

Interservice Physician Assistant Program
Special focus: Military Personnel Only
Location: Fort Sam Houston, TX
Degree granted: Master's Degree
Phone: 210-221-8004
E-mail: ipap@usarec.army.mil
Website: http://www.usarec.army.mil/armypa/
Supplemental application: Yes
Number of students accepted into program each year: N/A
Average GPA: >3.0
GRE: No
Length of program: 24 months
Uses CASPA: No
Tuition Cost: No cost – the program is free for selected students

Index of Residencies and Fellowships

Below, I have researched and listed the current PA residencies and fellowships. However, for the most current list of available PA residencies and fellowships, please review online at: http://www.appap.org/index1.html.

Cardiothoracic Surgery

1. The Methodist DeBaker Heart Center, Houston Texas
   Contact Person: Boris Bratovich
   Phone: 713-441-6201 or 713-790-2089
   E-mail: borisbratovich@sbcglobal.net

2. North Shore University Hospital, Manhasset, New York
   Contact Person: Bruce Hormann
   Phone: 516-562-4970
   E-mail: bhormann@nshs.edu

3. St. Joseph Mercy Hospital, Grand Rapids, Michigan
   Contact Person: Kristen Norris
   Phone: 734-712-7202
   E-mail: pasrp@spectrum-health.org or
   Kristen.snyder@devoschildrens.org

Critical Care

1. Oregon Health and Sciences University, Portland, Oregon
   Contact Person: Amy Juve
   Phone: 503-494-7641
   E-mail: juvea@ohsu.edu
   Website: http://www.ohsu.edu/anesth/recruitment/PA.htm

Dermatology

1. University of Texas Southwestern Medical Center, Dallas, Texas
   Contact Person: Jo Urquhart
   Phone: 214-648-8806
   E-mail: jo.urquhart@utsouthwestern.edu or
   eugene.jones@utsouthwestern.edu

Emergency Medicine

1. Johns Hopkins Bayview Medical Center, Baltimore, Maryland
    Contact Person: Jonathan Lerner
    Phone: 410-550-7911
    E-mail: paerres@jhmi.edu
    Website: http://www.hopkinsbayview.org/emresidency/index.html

2. Medical College of Georgia, Augusta, Georgia
    Contact Person: Yvonne Booker
    Phone: 706-721-2613
    E-mail: ybooker@mail.mcg.edu or boswald@mail.mcg.edu

3. University of Texas Health Science Center, San Antonio, Texas
    Contact Person: Peter Forsberg
    Phone: 210-358-2078/0636
    E-mail: forsbergp@uthscsa.edu

4. United States Army Medical Department, Fort Sam Houston, Texas
    Contact Person: Major Leonard Gruppo
    Phone: 210-916-3598
    E-mail: leonard.gruppo@amedd.army.mil

5. Wright Patterson, Wright Patterson Air Force Base, Ohio
    Contact Person: Captain Jim Garman
    Phone: 937-257-9259/0770
    E-mail:James.Garman@wpafb.af.mil or
    Timothy.bonjour@wpafb.af.mil

Hospitalist

1. Alderson-Broaddus College, Philippi, West Virginia
    Contact Person: William A. Childers
    Phone: 304-457-6356
    E-mail: childerswa@mail.ab.edu
    Website: http://www.ab.edu/academics/degrees/postgraduate

2. Mayo Clinic Arizona, Phoenix, Arizona
    Contact Person: Kristen Will or Zachary Hartsell
    Phone: 480-342-1387
    E-mail: will.kristen@mayo.edu or hartsell.zachary@mayo.edu
    Website: http://www.mayo.edu/mshs/pa-him-sct.html

Neonatology

1. University of Kentucky, Lexington, Kentucky
    Contact Person: Eric Reynolds
    Phone: 859-323-5530
    E-mail: ereyn2@uky.edu

Neurology

1. Neurological Associates of Northeastern New York, Schenectady, New York
    Contact Person: Victor G. Bruce
    Phone: 518-381-6042
    E-mail: vgbruce@aol.com

Neurosurgery

1. University of Arizona, Tucson, Arizona
    Contact Person: Martin Weinand
    Phone: 520-626-0704
    E-mail: mweinand@email.arizona.edu

Ob-Gyn

1. Riverside-Arrowhead Regional Medical Center, Colton, California
    Contact Person: Christine Sims
    Phone: 909-580-6320
    E-mail: Cervenkaj@ARMC.sbcounty.gov

Oncology

1. MD Anderson Cancer Center, Houston, Texas
    Contact Person: Maura Polansky
    Phone: 713-794-5002
    E-mail: paponc@mdanderson.org

Orthopaedic Surgery

1. Arrowhead Regional Medical Center, Colton, California
    Contact Person: Julie Mabry
    Phone: 909-580-6353/6330
    E-mail: N/A

2. Illinois Bone and Joint Institute, North Chicago, Illinois
    Contact Person: Patrick Knott
    Phone: 847-578-8689/8302
    E-mail: patrick.knott@rosalindfranklin.edu
    Website: http://www.rosalindfranklin.edu/srhs/passt/ortho.cfm

3. NYU Hospital for Joint Diseases, New York, New York
    Contact Person: Brian Donocoff
    Phone: 212-598-6497
    E-mail: brian.donocoff@med.nyu.edu

4. University of Florida, Jacksonville, Florida
    Contact Person: Michael Seese
    Phone: 904-633-0150
    E-mail: michael.seese@jax.ufl.edu

5. Watauga Orthopedics, Johnson City, Tennessee
    Contact Person: Robert Rogan
    Phone: (423) 282-9011
    E-mail: roganrb@wtodocs.com
    Website: www.Wataugaortho.com

Psychiatry

1. Cherokee Mental Health Institute, Cherokee, Iowa
    Contact Person: Daniel W. Gillette
    Phone: 712-225-2594
    E-mail: dgillet@dhs.state.ia.us or bdirks@dhs.state.ia.us

2. University of Iowa Behavioral Health, Iowa City, Iowa
    Contact Person: Don St. John
    Phone: 319-353-6314
    E-mail: don-stjohn@uiowa.edu

Rheumatology

1. University of Texas Southwestern at Dallas, Dallas, Texas
    Contact Person: Cheryl Bedford
    Phone: 214-648-3969
    E-mail: Cheryl.Bedford@UTSouthwestern.edu

Surgery

1. Alderson-Broaddus College, Philippi, West Virginia
    Contact Person: William A. Childers
    Phone: 304-457-6356
    E-mail: childerswa@mail.ab.edu
    Website: http://www.ab.edu/academics/degrees/postgraduate

2. Arrowhead Regional Medical Center, Colton, California
    Contact Person: Victor Joe
    Phone: 909-580-6210
    E-mail: joev@armc.sbcounty.gov

3. Bassett Healthcare, Cooperstown, New York
    Contact Person: Shari Johnson-Ploutz
    Phone: 607-547-6672
    E-mail: shari.johnson-ploutz@bassett.org
    Website: http://www.bassett.org/edu/index.cfm

4. Duke University Medical Center, Durham, North Carolina
    Contact Person: Alicia M. Brown
    Phone: 919-684-2705
    E-mail: cynthia.cayton@duke.edu

5. Geisinger Medical Center, Danville, Pennsylvania
    Contact Person: Melissa Sedor
    Phone: 570-271-6361
    E-mail: mesedor@geisinger.edu

6. Grand Rapids PA Surgical Residency, Grand Rapids, Michigan
    Contact Person: Kristen Norris
    Phone: 616-391-8651
    E-mail: pasrp@spectrum-health.org or
    Kristen.snyder@devoschildrens.org

7. The Johns Hopkins Hospital, Baltimore, Maryland
    Contact Person: G. Melville Williams
    Phone: 443-622-2495
    E-mail: pasurgres@jhmi.edu
    Website: http://www.hopkinsmedicine.org/surgery/education/
    pa_residency/index.html

8. Montefiore Medical Center, Bronx, New York
    Contact Person: N/A
    Phone: 718-920-6223
    E-mail: N/A
    Website: http://www.montefiore.org/prof/residency/
    physician_assistant_interns/

9. The Hospital of Central Connecticut, New Britain, Connecticut
    Contact Person: Richard L. Commaille
    Phone: 860-224-5513
    E-mail: rconte@nbgh.org

10. Norwalk Hospital/Yale University of Medicine, Norwalk, Connecticut
    Contact Person: Virginia O. Hilton
    Phone: 203-852-2188
    E-mail: surpares@norwalkhealth.org

11. Medical College of Wisconsin, Milwaukee, Wisconsin
    Contact Person: K. Somers
    Phone: 414-266-6593
    E-mail: surgeryed@mcw.edu

Trauma/ Critical Care

1. Bridgeport Hospital, Bridgeport, Connecticut
   Contact Person: Paul Possenti
   Phone: 203-384-4598
   E-mail: ppposs@bpthospital.org

2. St. Luke's Hospital, Bethlehem, Pennsylvania
   Contact Person: Laurie N. Wilson
   Phone: 610-954-2207
   E-mail: wilsonla@slhn.org

Urology

1. Northwest Metropolitan Urology Associates, Park Ridge, Illinois
   Contact Person: Brian Hennig
   Phone: 773-775-0800
   E-mail: hennig01@comcast.net

Teaching Fellowships:

1. Medical University of South Carolina, Charleston, South Carolina
   Contact Person: Glen Askins
   Phone: 843-792-1913
   E-mail: askinsdg@musc.edu
   Website: http://www.musc.edu/chp/pa/Fellow/index.htm

2. Duke University Medical Center, Durham, North Carolina
   Contact Person: Karen J. Hills
   Phone: 919-668-6400
   E-mail: karen.hills@duke.edu
   Website: http://paprogram.mc.duke.edu/s_postgrad_tf.asp

3. Rosalind Franklin University, North Chicago, Illinois
    Contact Person: Patrick Knott
    Phone: 847-578-8302
    E-mail: Patrick.Knott@RosalindFranklin.edu
    Website: http://www.rosalindfranklin.edu/teachingfellowship.cfm.

Index

References

Accreditation Review Commission on Education for the Physician Assistant. Available at: http:// www.arc-pa.org. Accessed December 20, 2007.

American Academy of Nurse Practitioners. Available at: http://www.aanp.org/Default.asp. Accessed December 20, 2007.

American Academy of Physician Assistants. Available at: http://www.aapa.org. Accessed December 20, 2007.

American Association of Surgical Physician Assistants. Available at: http://www.aaspa.com. Accessed December 20, 2007.

American College of Physicians Position paper: physician assistants and nurse practitioners. Ann Intern Med. 1994; 121:714-716.

American Medical Association. Available at: http://www.ama-assn.org. Accessed December 20, 2007.

American Nurses Association. Available at: http://www.ana.org. Accessed December 20, 2007.

Association of Family Practice Physician Assistants. Available at: http://www.afppa.org. Accessed December 20, 2007.

Association of Postgraduate Physician Assistant Programs. Available at: http://www.appap.org/index1.html. Accessed December 20, 2007.

Bolles R. What Color Is Your Parachute? A Practical Manual for Job-Hunters and Career-Changers. Ten Speed Press, 2006.

Center for Disease Control: HIPAA Privacy Rule and Public Health. Available at: http://www.cdc.gov/mmwr/preview/mmwrhtml/su5201a1.htm. Accessed December 20, 2007.

Centers for Medicare and Medicaid Services - HIPPA General Information. Available at: http://www.cms.hhs.gov/HIPAAGenInfo. Accessed December 20, 2007.

CNN Money: 50 Best Jobs in America. Available at: http://money.cnn.com/magazines/moneymag/moneymag_archive/2006/05/01/8375749/index.htm. Accessed December 20, 2007.

Cooper RA, Laud P, Dietrich CL. Current and Projected Workforce of Nonphysician Clinicians. JAMA. 1998; 280:9,788-794.

References

Dehn R. Impending health workforce shortages and implications for PAs. Available at: http://jaapa.com/issues/j20061201/articles/guestedit1206.htm. Accessed December 20, 2007.

DeWalch, D. The Surgical Physician Assistant: Practice Reimbursement and Utilization Handbook. American Association of Surgical Physician Assistants Publishing; 2006.

Druss, et al. Trends in care by non-physician clinicians in the U.S. The New England Journal of Medicine. 2003;348:130-7.

Get Into Medical School: A Strategic Approach (Get Into Medical School). Kaplan Publishing. 2006.

Miller R, Bissell D. Med School Confidential: A Complete Guide to the Medical School Experience: By Students, for Students. St. Martin's Griffin Publisher. 2006.

Mittman DE, Cawley JF, Fenn WH. Physician Assistants in the United States. British Medical Journal. 2002;325:7362,485-487.

National Commission on Certification of Physician Assistants. Available at: http://www.nccpa.net. Accessed December 20, 2007.

National Organization of Nurse Practitioner Faculties. Available at: http://www.nonpf.org. Accessed December 20, 2007.

O'Reilly K. Medicare plans to stop paying for 6 hospital-acquired conditions. Available at: http://www.ama-assn.org/amednews/2007/06/18/gvsb0618.htm. Accessed December 20, 2007.

Physician Assistant Education Association. Available at: http://www.paeaonline.org/index.html. Accessed December 20, 2007.

Physician Assistant History Center. Available at: http://www.pahx.org/index.htm. Accessed December 20, 2007.

Robyn E. Mitchell: Evaluating The Clinical Preparation Of Physician Assistant Versus Nurse Practitioner Students And The Characteristics Of Their Preceptors. The Internet Journal of Academic Physician Assistants. 2004. Volume 4 Number 1. Available at: http://www.ispub.com/ostia/index.php?xmlFilePath=journals/ijapa/vol4n1/mhe.xml. Accessed December 20, 2007.

Rodican A. Getting Into the PA School of Your Choice, Second Edition. McGraw-Hill Medical. 2003.

Student Academy of the American Academy of Physician Assistants. Available at: http://saaapa.aapa.org/index.htm. Accessed December 20, 2007.

U.S. Department of Labor: Bureau of Labor Statistics. Available at: http://stats.bls.gov/oco/ocos081.htm. Accessed December 20, 2007.

United States Department of Health and Human Services- CMS. Available at: http://www.cms.hhs.gov/transmittals/downloads/R1734B3.pdf. Accessed December 20, 2007.

Wisconsin Program for Training Regionally Employed Care Providers (WisTREC). Available at: http://academic.son.wisc.edu/wistrec. Accessed December 20, 2007.

About the Author

Erin Sherer is a physician assistant and dietitian currently living and working in Michigan. She received her Bachelor of Science degree in dietetics from Michigan State University, her Physician Assistant Certificate from the Weill Medical College of Cornell University, and her Master of Physician Assistant Studies Degree from the University of Nebraska Medical Center. She enjoys working with physician assistant students as well as helping to promote the PA profession.

1859687